# HENRY DANIEL AND THE RISE OF MIDDLE ENGLISH MEDICAL WRITING

EDITED BY SARAH STAR

# Henry Daniel and the Rise of Middle English Medical Writing

UNIVERSITY OF TORONTO PRESS
Toronto Buffalo London

© University of Toronto Press 2022
Toronto Buffalo London
utorontopress.com

ISBN 978-1-4875-2953-6 (cloth)    ISBN 978-1-4875-2955-0 (EPUB)
                                  ISBN 978-1-4875-2954-3 (PDF)

---

**Library and Archives Canada Cataloguing in Publication**

Title: Henry Daniel and the rise of Middle English medical writing / edited by
    Sarah Star.
Names: Star, Sarah, editor.
Description: Includes bibliographical references and index.
Identifiers: Canadiana (print) 20210293365 | Canadiana (ebook) 20210294353 |
    ISBN 9781487529536 (hardcover) | ISBN 9781487529550 (EPUB) |
    ISBN 9781487529543 (PDF)
Subjects: LCSH: Daniel, Henry (Medical writer) | LCSH: Medicine, Medieval –
    England. | LCSH: Medical writing – History – To 1500. | LCSH: Medical
    literature – England – History – To 1500. | LCSH: England – Intellectual
    life – 1066–1485.
Classification: LCC R141 .H46 2022 | DDC 610.942/09023–dc23

---

We wish to acknowledge the land on which the University of Toronto Press
operates. This land is the traditional territory of the Wendat, the Anishnaabeg,
the Haudenosaunee, the Métis, and the Mississaugas of the Credit First Nation.

University of Toronto Press gratefully acknowledges the financial assistance
of the Centre for Medieval Studies, University of Toronto in the publication of
this book.

University of Toronto Press acknowledges the financial support of the
Government of Canada, the Canada Council for the Arts, and the Ontario Arts
Council, an agency of the Government of Ontario, for its publishing activities.

Canada Council     Conseil des Arts
for the Arts       du Canada

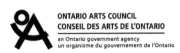

ONTARIO ARTS COUNCIL
CONSEIL DES ARTS DE L'ONTARIO

an Ontario government agency
un organisme du gouvernement de l'Ontario

Funded by the    Financé par le
Government       gouvernement
of Canada        du Canada

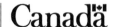

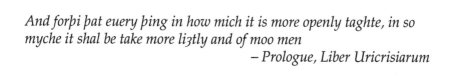

*And forþi þat euery þing in how mich it is more openly taghte, in so myche it shal be take more liȝtly and of moo men*
— *Prologue, Liber Uricrisiarum*

# Contents

# Preface

This edited collection was conceived as part of the ongoing Henry Daniel Project based at the University of Toronto (https://henrydaniel.utoronto.ca/), which aims to edit and publish Daniel's works and stimulate new scholarship on them. The Social Sciences and Humanities Research Council of Canada has provided substantial support for the projects that initiated this volume, including the publication of the *Liber Uricrisiarum: A Reading Edition*, the current work towards an edition of Henry Daniel's herbal treatise, and the 52nd Conference on Editorial Problems held at the Centre for Medieval Studies at the University of Toronto in 2017. For the permissions to use the image that appears on the cover of this volume (Gloucester, Cathedral Library, MS 19, f. 27r), I thank archivist Rebecca Phillips. The illustration exemplifies the topic of this volume: reading Henry Daniel. Added to the medieval manuscript by its owner Henry Fowler in the seventeenth century, the illustration captures one reader's enthusiastic response.

The volume changed throughout the past few years, with new contributions and some rethinking, and I benefitted from the advice of many colleagues along the way. For sharing her unedited transcriptions of Daniel's *Liber Uricrisiarum* and herbal manual with other contributors, and for introducing me to Henry Daniel in the first place, I owe my greatest thanks to E. Ruth Harvey. For his role getting this volume started and for his contributions in the beginning, I'd like to thank Nicholas Everett. For her ongoing editorial guidance, for taking the lead creating the *Liber Uricrisiarum* content guide appendix, and for offering her keen eye, I heartily thank M. Teresa Tavormina. For providing invaluable advice and useful perspectives, I thank Suzanne Conklin Akbari, David Townsend, and Anna Wilson. The staff at the University of Toronto Press, especially Suzanne Rancourt and Barb Porter, have supported this volume since its initial stages and facilitated a smooth and enjoyable production process, for which I'm very grateful. I would also like to thank Jeff Espie for his unwavering support, both personal and professional.

# Sigils of Witnesses

## The *Liber Uricrisiarum* and Its Adaptations

| | |
|---|---|
| A | Oxford, Bodleian Library, Ashmole MS 1404 |
| B | Boston, Massachusetts Historical Society, MS P-361 (*olim* 10.10) |
| Br | Brussels, Bibliothèque Royale, MS IV.249 (now in private hands) |
| Cf | Cambridge, University Library, MS Ff.2.6 |
| Cg | Cambridge, University Library, MS Gg.3.29 |
| E | London, British Library, Egerton MS 1624 |
| G | Gloucester, Cathedral Library MS 19 |
| G3 | Cambridge, Gonville and Caius College Library, MS 180/213 |
| G5 | Cambridge, Gonville and Caius College Library, MS 336/725 |
| G6 | Cambridge, Gonville and Caius College Library, MS 376/596 |
| G7 | Cambridge, Gonville and Caius College Library, MS 176/97 |
| H | San Marino, Huntington Library, MS HM 505 |
| Hu | Glasgow, University Library, Hunterian MS 328 |
| J | Cambridge, St John's College Library, MS B.16 |
| Jt | New York, Jewish Theological Seminary of America, MS 2611 |
| Ju | *The Iudycyall of Vryns* (Southwark: P. Treveris, ?1527) |
| L | Glasgow, University Library, Hunterian MS 362 |
| L6 | Oxford, Bodleian Library, lat.misc. MS c.66 |
| M6 | Oxford, Bodleian Library, e Musaeo MS 116 |
| M7 | Oxford, Bodleian Library, e Musaeo MS 187 |
| P | London, Royal College of Physicians, MS 356 |
| Pe | Cambridge, Magdalene College Library, Pepys MS 1661 |
| R | London, British Library, Royal MS 17 D.i |
| Ra | Oxford, Bodleian Library, Rawlinson MS D.1221 |
| Sa | London, British Library, Sloane MS 1100 |
| Sb | London, British Library, Sloane MS 1101 |
| Sc | London, British Library, Sloane MS 1721 |

Sd    London, British Library, Sloane MS 1088
Se    London, British Library, Sloane MS 2527
Sf    London, British Library, Sloane MS 134
Sg    London, British Library, Sloane MS 2196
Sh    London, British Library, Sloane MS 5
Si    London, British Library, Sloane MS 340
T     Cambridge, Trinity College Library, MS O.10.21
T2    Cambridge, Trinity College Library, MS R.14.52
W     London, Wellcome Library, MS 225
W6    London, Wellcome Library, MS 226
W7    London, Wellcome Library, MS 7117
Y     New Haven, Yale Medical School, Cushing-Whitney Library
      MS 45


**Daniel's Herbal**

Add    London, British Library, Additional MS 27329
Ar     London, British Library, Arundel MS 42

# HENRY DANIEL AND THE RISE OF MIDDLE ENGLISH MEDICAL WRITING

*Introduction*

# Reading Henry Daniel

SARAH STAR

Henry Daniel, a fourteenth-century Dominican friar, wrote two impressive academic medical treatises in Middle English, the significance of which modern scholarship has only barely begun to grasp: first, the *Liber Uricrisiarum* (ca. 1375–82), a diagnostic text on uroscopy, and then, shortly after, an herbal manual.[1] Composing medical texts in English during the last quarter of the fourteenth century was rare, and doing so places Daniel on the cusp of what would become a burgeoning vernacular movement. He tells "Walter Turnour of Ketoun" (Pro.5),[2] his colleague and commissioner of the *Liber Uricrisiarum*, about the text's originality. Daniel asserts himself as the first to write uroscopy in English: "I haue redde ne harde neyþer þis science giffen in English" (Pro.13). In asking him to write this English treatise, Walter has consequently, Daniel explains, "put me to an harde wark and opne to the barking & to the scornyng of detractours" (Pro.9–10). Literary critics deeply indebted to scholarship concerning Wycliffite vernacularization might view such statements about the "scornyng of detractours" as highly politicised, indicative of the potential heretical association of translating the authoritative knowledge typically written exclusively in Latin.[3] The political stakes of biblical translation, for instance, came to a head in the first decade of the fifteenth century with the Constitutions of Archbishop Thomas Arundel, which restricted the translation of Scripture and regulated preaching and the production and use of vernacular books. The risks associated with Lollard endeavours, however, do not provide a complete framework through which to understand the English translation and vernacularization of other, "authoritative" discourses.

Medicine is just such an authoritative discourse – one that can achieve, as Daniel seems to celebrate in his Prologue, a new prominence in English rather than a (yet un-thought of) Arundelian circumscription. In her foundational work on medieval textual cultures, Linda Ehrsam Voigts has shown that the late fourteenth century marks the beginning of Middle English medicine, a field that would undergo "rapid growth" over the next hundred years. Voigts's collaborative *eVK* database, for example, catalogues several thousand Middle English manuscript witnesses to medical and scientific texts.[4] The records of extant medical and scientific manuscripts indicate that knowledge previously reserved for (or translated into) Latin began trickling into the vernacular around 1375, ultimately giving rise to an explosion of Middle English medicine in the fifteenth century.[5] Though Daniel could not have predicted this forthcoming boom, he nevertheless makes a self-conscious claim as the originator of one vernacular medical tradition: uroscopy.

According to Daniel, writing uroscopy in English will increase access to this important knowledge. Daniel explains that he composes his treatise "noȝt for cause of lucre of fauour as oþer men doþ" (Pro.36–7). Instead, he elucidates, "charite broght me more herto þan hardines" (Pro.88). Daniel's insistence that he does not seek financial gain remains thoroughly in keeping with his theological position. As the scholarship on medieval friar physicians has demonstrated, friars who wrote or practised medicine did so, like Daniel, out of charity.[6] Daniel stands alone, however, in the scope of his benevolence. His charitable impulse, indicated by his desire to be "profitable vnto men" (Pro.44–5), aims at healing the bodies of the sick, but it also involves expanding all minds. The treatise aspires to make uroscopy "more openly taghte" (Pro.47) so that it may, in turn, "be take[n] more liȝtly & of moo men" (Pro.47–8). Daniel writes the *Liber Uricrisiarum* with consideration for the many people who, he thinks, "couaiteþ to be experte of demyng of vrines" (Pro.42–3). His charity, rather than being limited to his provision of individual diagnoses, involves his gift of the diagnostic power itself. Daniel aims to increase access to uroscopic knowledge and, in doing so, to help people learn uroscopy for themselves.

The present volume aims to extend Daniel's project. Both the *Liber Uricrisiarum* and the herbal have a studiously encyclopaedic scope; but, despite their own learnedness, neither has received much modern scholarly attention. The essays compiled here seek to introduce scholars from a wide range of disciplines – medieval medicine, history of medicine and science, intellectual history, philology, history of English, vernacularization, lexicology, manuscript studies, medieval religious studies, and Middle English literary studies – to Daniel's work. His representation of science, religion, and language might influence a wide array of critical fields; and this volume accordingly shows several scholarly conversations for which Daniel might matter. The essay collection also serves as a critical companion to the recently published *Liber Uricrisiarum: A Reading Edition*, the first complete edition of Daniel's uroscopy treatise.[7] The edition presents a complete version of the text and provides a detailed introduction to Daniel's life and work as well as to the manuscripts used for the edition. The companion explains the authoritative background of Daniel's uroscopic and herbal work, his relationship to his sources, and his originality; it describes all known versions of the *Liber Uricrisiarum* and traces revisions over time; it analyses Daniel's representations of his own medical practice; and it demonstrates his influence on later medical and literary writers. I and my fellow contributors hope that this collection will make Daniel's texts "more openly taghte" and prompt new scholarship on their significance.

## A New Authority

Daniel wrote the *Liber Uricrisiarum* in Latin first, and then translated his own text into English. The English Prologue outlines the process, as Daniel explains that he has "gadrede now late for þam þat kan take it in Latyn a schorte tretice conteynyng fully þe marowe of þis faculte" (Pro.79–81).[8] By telling his readers that he has written his uroscopic material in English and in Latin, Daniel reveals a relationship to his sources more multifaceted than previous scholars have acknowledged. Until recently, the scholarly tendency has been to claim Daniel's *Liber Uricrisiarum* as a translation of a translation: an English translation of Constantine the African's Latin translation of Isaac Judaeus's *De urinis*. According to Joanne Jasin, for instance, Daniel's *Liber Uricrisiarum* can be considered a translation of *De urinis* based on Daniel's own authority.[9] To be sure, Isaac's work exerts a major influence on Daniel. As Jasin points out, Daniel states that he provides a translation of Isaac's *De urinis* "nerhande worde for worde." Jasin assigns this declaration, however, a wider applicability than Daniel himself allows; he uses its phrasing to denote not the treatise in its entirety but only a few chapters of it.[10] E. Ruth Harvey and M. Teresa Tavormina demonstrate in their introduction to the *Liber Uricrisiarum* in the recent edition, by contrast, that Daniel modelled his own text on the framework of Gilles de Corbeil. They discuss, moreover, his many other influences in detail, including Galen, Hippocrates, and Theophilus, as well as Isaac.[11] Rather than translating *De urinis* in isolation, Daniel's English treatise is – as he notes in its Prologue – a vernacular rendering of his own Latin work, one that he compiled using a combination of learned sources.

Faith Wallis's chapter in this volume develops the preliminary work of Harvey and Tavormina. Outlining the Latin uroscopic tradition from which Daniel draws his information, Wallis argues for the "uniquely significant role of urine science in western medicine." She focuses on four important Latin texts (Theophilus's *De urinis*, Isaac Judaeus's *De urinis*, Gilles de Corbeil's *Carmen de urinis*, and Avicenna's *Canon*), and demonstrates the crucial role of urine science in both medical theory and medical practice. The urine science that Daniel inherits from his Latin sources, she shows, thus distinctively served two purposes at once. Since urine signified the inner workings of the body, theorizing the science also "carried in its wake the need to make that science usable by practitioners." Daniel similarly finds his place within an existing Latin tradition in writing the herbal. In this case, as Winston Black demonstrates in his chapter, much of the authoritative material appears originally in verse. Its form requires Daniel to undertake a "process of double translation" as he adapts Latin material into English and verse into prose. Black argues that Daniel's double translation of two Latin sources in particular – the *De viribus herbarum* of Macer Floridus and the *Anglicanus Ortus* of Henry of Huntingdon – reveals a thoughtful process of selection. He chose which passages to translate carefully, which ideas to pass over, which to censor, and "which needed further explanation for his English audience."

Both chapters thoroughly explain Daniel's relationship to his authoritative sources, while also gesturing towards Daniel's own originality. Self-consciously positioning his work in relation to preceding traditions, Daniel claims in the Prologue to the *Liber Uricrisiarum* that he writes not "newe þinges" but "newely" (Pro.79). His diction suggests that the *Liber Uricrisiarum* may undertake its own project of translation, compilation, and adaptation, similar to that described by Black in the herbal. In addition to writing down in new form already existing medical ideas, Daniel also relies on his own experience for accurate information. After explaining in the Prologue that he has gathered knowledge from experts, such as those described in Wallis's chapter, Daniel adds that, "I lefte meny þingz or addede to myne owen þat som auctoures affermeth noȝt" (Pro.56–7). As opposed to writing only "newely," Daniel here asserts his inventiveness.[12] He advertises his omission of authoritative material with which he does not agree; and he highlights his addition of new ideas about uroscopy. By explaining this part of his compilation process, Daniel suggests that writing "newely" and writing "newe þinges" need not remain as mutually exclusive as he had earlier implied. The *Liber Uricrisiarum*, to be sure, is not an entirely original work; but neither does it comprise translated ideas alone. By writing "newely," Daniel grants himself an intellectual licence. He chooses just how much authoritative knowledge he will transmit; and he strives in the process to establish his treatise as a vernacular uroscopic authority in its own right. If Daniel allows a pre-existing body of specialised knowledge to be "more openly taghte," he also decides what this new pedagogical programme will entail.

Daniel's originality appears not only in his relationship to his Latin sources, but also in his connection with his English contemporaries. Peter Murray Jones builds on the chapters by Wallis and Black by analysing Daniel within his contemporary medical context, alongside other English authorities, such as John Arderne, John Mirfield, John Bradmore, and Gilbert Kymer, and other friars, such as William Holme. Jones demonstrates that Daniel's "project was different from theirs in important ways," including in its intended audience, its medical interest, and its language of composition (Daniel's English contemporaries wrote exclusively in Latin). Their differences notwithstanding, contemporary medical texts, Jones contends, can still illuminate the significance of Daniel's English contribution. His work "shares their preoccupation" with teaching complex medical material. Read alongside his contemporaries, Daniel proves himself both "a member of this extraordinary generation" of English medical writers, as well as a distinct individual within it.

Daniel's texts show remarkable, multilingual learning, even if his audience may not have shared it. His compilation of uroscopic and herbal knowledge in English, after all, only serves its full intention if his intended readers could not simply turn to the Latin authorities themselves. As Daniel explains in the Prologue to the *Liber Uricrisiarum*, his Latin treatise addresses "þam þat kan take it." The expanded English version, meanwhile, presents its knowledge for unlettered "ydiotes" (Pro.29) – people who cannot read Latin, who want to practise medicine but lack the fundamentals. In his own words, Daniel writes the English treatise "considerand meny men & diuerse þat couaiteþ to be experte of demyng of vrines" (Pro.42–3). Harvey and Tavormina likewise suggest in their introduction to *A Reading Edition* that Daniel's audience could have comprised a wide array of people, not all of whom would have access to his Latin sources. "He wants to use the best authorities," they explain, "and to make them available to an audience which must have included many of the kinds of people Daniel had met in his life." Daniel encountered a literate gentry, apothecaries and herbalists, physicians, and travellers. He may have equally addressed "intelligent but illiterate folk who could afford to have someone read to them" – people similar to "his various informants, who had practiced 'medicine' of a sort at all levels of society."[13] Daniel aims, in short, to compose texts in which impressive learning becomes widely accessible.

## Manuscripts, Editions, and Texts

Though linguistically and intellectually accessible in his own time, Daniel's texts have not always remained readily available to modern readers; scholarship on Daniel has yet to register his full importance, predominantly due to a problem of limited publication. The herbal has never appeared in a modern edition, in part because its text presents major editorial challenges.[14] It survives in two manuscripts, each representing a distinct version of the treatise.[15] The *Liber Uricrisiarum* has received only slightly more publicity. In 1983, Joanne Jasin transcribed one manuscript of the text for an edition that would comprise her dissertation.[16] Similarly, in 2005, Tom Johannessen transcribed another manuscript for his master's thesis.[17] Meanwhile, in 1994, Ralph Hanna edited the English Prologue and the first three chapters from Book 1.[18] Hanna's partial edition reached a wider scholarly audience than either Jasin's dissertation or Johannessen's thesis, and it includes an important introduction as well as detailed explanatory notes. As a short excerpt, however, it necessarily omits the vast majority of Daniel's text. All complete versions of the *Liber Uricrisiarum* contain three books, even if the number of chapters changes from one manuscript version to the next. The version used for *A Reading Edition*, edited by Harvey, Tavormina, and Star (University of Toronto Press, 2020) has four chapters in Book 1, fourteen in Book 2, and twenty in Book 3, and provides the basis for the first complete edition of Daniel's uroscopy. A full critical edition still awaits.[19]

While the herbal survives in two manuscripts, each representing a discrete version, the *Liber Uricrisiarum* has more overlap in its various texts. Daniel's uroscopy appears extant in thirty-seven manuscripts and two print copies, all of which have, as Harvey and Tavormina outline in their introduction to *A Reading Edition*, a complex relationship.[20] Harvey develops that introduction substantially in her chapter included here. Based on her extensive archival research, she outlines for the *Liber Uricrisiarum* several "textual layers." She explains that there are at least five versions of the text: the two main versions she calls the "alpha" and the "beta"; the other three are the "proto-alpha," the "first revision," and the "beta star." Harvey categorises the manuscripts according to what dates they include internally, what contents they contain or omit, and how they represent certain medical details. As she notes, attempting to sort out the entire textual history across each manuscript presents "an enormous task." Far from giving the final word on the text's complicated history, Harvey provides a description at once coherent and liable to change – the most comprehensive account to date of the manuscripts' varied connections. She also shows in unprecedented detail the major subjects of Daniel's revisions, such as his discussions of astronomy and his consideration of women's health. In doing so, Harvey's chapter enables future work on Daniel in particular and on medieval revision practices more generally. Daniel's revisionary practice may prove especially useful as a point of comparison for William Langland's *Piers Plowman*. Likewise adapting Latin learning into the English language, Langland revised his three versions of *Piers* contemporaneously with Daniel's revisions to the *Liber*.[21]

In revising the text over time, Daniel provides varying degrees of detail on his own medical practice. In both the *Liber Uricrisiarum* and the herbal, Daniel occasionally describes his participation in or observation of his contemporary medical community, which, as I have demonstrated elsewhere, comprises people "both learned and lay."[22] He comments on experiences he has had with apothecaries and physicians as well as with neighbours and gossips, representing his medical world as "a whole network of advisers, lay and expert, men and women."[23] Daniel's revisionary practice in the *Liber Uricrisiarum* means, however, that different audiences had access to different stories about illness and diagnosis. The version of the text published in *A Reading Edition*, for instance, includes only one case history, whereas other manuscripts include three others. Hannah Bower's chapter in this volume quotes all case histories at length, and so gives readers access to textual details beyond what *A Reading Edition* allows. In these histories, as Bower argues, Daniel uses narrative techniques such as deferral, suspense, and plot twists, all of which recall "more literary writings." His narrative mode not only makes for surprising endings, but also de-centres "inadequate medical authorities" and decreases the conventional emphasis on sight. Whereas traditional medical practice stresses the importance of sight to uroscopic diagnosis, Bower suggests that Daniel uses narrative to privilege a multitude of voices and argue for the relevance of hearing different stories.

## Daniel's Literary and Medical Heirs

Daniel's understanding of medicine as a communal, multivocal endeavour is reflected in the early reception history of the *Liber Uricrisiarum*. In her chapter, M. Teresa Tavormina outlines that history in detail. Tavormina's archival research shows that Daniel's *Liber Uricrisiarum* ranks in the "top five most frequently copied and/or reworked Middle English uroscopies," meaning that excerpts, abridgments, and adaptations occur in several manuscripts throughout the fifteenth and sixteenth centuries.[24] Her chapter surveys all of the reworkings found to date, identifying the manuscripts in which they occur and analysing the kinds of changes they make. Tavormina organises her argument according to the relationship between Daniel's original work and its reworking: citations, short excerpts, supplements, extracts and abridgments of individual books, and adaptations of the full text. The chapter as a whole demonstrates that the *Liber Uricrisiarum* circulated in a wide array of new forms throughout the fifteenth and sixteenth centuries: Daniel's early vernacular work had a lasting importance. Scholarship often measures the success or popularity of a medieval text by the number of its extant manuscripts; as Tavormina shows, however, doing so only tells part of a text's history in the world. Here, she aims to present a fuller picture of the *Liber Uricrisiarum*'s afterlife and to show the many functions that its text could serve.

The afterlife of Daniel's work extends beyond medical discourse alone. As a medical writer aiming to make uroscopic science available to English readers, Daniel necessarily had to expand the English language itself. Over a thousand words from one manuscript of the *Liber Uricrisiarum*, for example, predate or emerge with their earliest cited occurrences in the *Middle English Dictionary* and *Oxford English Dictionary*. Daniel made a considerable contribution to Middle English and its significance warrants further attention.[25] Daniel participated, after all, in a larger project of fourteenth-century vernacularization, alongside other linguistic innovators, such as Langland, Gower, and Chaucer.[26] As I show in my chapter, in fact, his *Liber Uricrisiarum* comprises "as much a treatise *on* English as *in* English." I focus here on what Daniel calls his "almost-Latin" words – English/Latin hybrids – and demonstrate how Daniel's linguistic innovations inform his distinctly vernacular style. I also show that his creative, hybrid language forms for Daniel a literary legacy that extends beyond direct influence alone. Many Latinate terms that appear first in Daniel surface again, several decades later, in John Lydgate's *Fabula duorum mercatorum*, a fifteenth-century poem that includes a meaningful discussion of uroscopy as well. Sharing many of Daniel's new terms, the *Fabula* develops in English a specifically medical poetics, and constructs a history for linguistic "aureation" that exceeds the more familiar past of Chaucerian eloquence.

These two chapters exemplify a commitment central to this volume as a whole, which demonstrates Daniel's relevance for both multiple premodern traditions and multiple modern disciplines. The *Liber Uricrisiarum* and the herbal hold substantial significance in the studies of medieval medicine and uroscopic science, as Faith Wallis demonstrates; of medieval pharmacology and translation, as Winston Black shows;

of medieval English medical communities and mendicant writings, as Peter Murray Jones explains; of textual transmission and authorial revision, as E. Ruth Harvey argues; of textual reception and readerly adaptation, as M. Teresa Tavormina illustrates; of narrative technique and sensory perception, as Hannah Bower reveals; and of literary style and linguistic innovation, as I suggest. The essays in this volume thus demonstrate that "Reading Henry Daniel" makes it possible to think capaciously – to think about uroscopies and herbals as at the centre of multiple branches of study.

*A Note on Citations*

We have aimed for as much consistency as possible regarding the citations of Daniel's texts. Most quotations from the text of the *Liber Uricrisiarum* are drawn from the edition by Harvey, Tavormina, and Star, and are consequently cited here by book, chapter, and line number in the edition (e.g., 2.4.11–13). When a contributor cites a passage that does not appear in the edition, they cite by manuscript shelf mark and folio number (e.g., London, British Library, Sloane MS 1088, f. 63r). An exception is E. Ruth Harvey's chapter. Since Harvey cites from so many manuscripts to illustrate the "textual layers" of the *Liber Uricrisiarum*, she cites by manuscript sigil and either book, chapter, and line number (e.g., R 1.3.14–16) or folio number (e.g., A, f. 55v), according to whether the passage appears in the edition or in a manuscript not used for the edition. Harvey provides the manuscript shelf mark for each sigil she uses; a complete list of sigils appears at xi–xii of the present volume.

Quotations from the herbal are cited by manuscript shelf mark and folio number (e.g., London, British Library, Additional MS 27329, f. 43r). When a contributor clarifies that they are citing from just one manuscript, only the first citation includes the manuscript shelf mark and all subsequent quotations provide only the folio number (e.g., 36v).

Quotations from all other manuscripts are cited by manuscript shelf mark and folio number.

NOTES

1  I and my fellow contributors refer to Daniel's herbal manual simply as "the herbal" throughout most of this volume. As Winston Black explains in his chapter, the text does not have a contemporary title. In one manuscript (London, British Library, Additional MS 27329), a later hand provides

*Aaron Danielis* as a title. Black's chapter focuses on that version of the herbal and therefore uses the title provided in the manuscript.

2  This and all quotations from the English Prologue to Henry Daniel's *Liber Uricrisiarum* are from *Liber Uricrisiarum: A Reading Edition*, edited by E. Ruth Harvey, M. Teresa Tavormina, and Sarah Star (Toronto: University of Toronto Press, 2020), hereafter cited parenthetically by line number.

3  See Fiona Somerset, *Clerical Discourse and Lay Audience in Late Medieval England* (Cambridge: Cambridge University Press, 1998) and Anne Hudson, *The Premature Reformation: Wycliffite Texts and Lollard History* (Oxford: Clarendon Press, 1988) and "The Debate on Bible Translation, Oxford 1401," *English Historical Review* XC. CCCLIV (1975): 1–18. Rita Copeland argues that the clergy-laity binary is more than one of Latin-vernacular and is based, instead, on an earlier association of the laity with the literal sense of Scripture. See *Pedagogy, Intellectuals, and Dissent in the Later Middle Ages: Lollardy and Ideas of Learning* (Cambridge: Cambridge University Press, 2001).

4  See Linda Ehrsam Voigts, "Multitudes of Middle English Manuscripts, or the Englishing of Science and Medicine" in Margaret R. Schleissner, ed., *Manuscript Sources of Medieval England: A Book of Essays* (New York and London: Garland Publishing, 1995), 183–96. As Voigts herself explains, these large numbers comprise both "scientific" and "medical" texts; the precise number of specifically "medical" texts, though substantial, is difficult to determine.

5  See Voigts, "Scientific and Medical Books" in Jeremy Griffiths and Derek Pearsall, ed., *Book Production and Publishing in Britain, 1375–1475* (Cambridge: Cambridge University Press, 1989), 345–402. Voigts here suggests that the period of 1375–1500 is partially "arbitrary," but also marks "a fairly well-defined period of increasing use of the vernacular for medical and scientific writing" (352). This period, indeed, is now used widely by medical historians, most notably Irma Taavitsainen and Päivi Pahta in "Vernacularisation of Scientific and Medical Writing in its Sociohistorical Context" in *Medical and Scientific Writing in Late Medieval English* (Cambridge: Cambridge University Press, 2004), 1–22. For information on extant Middle English uroscopies in particular, see M. Teresa Tavormina, "Uroscopy in Middle English: A Guide to the Texts and Manuscripts," *Studies in Medieval and Renaissance History*, 3rd series, 26:11 (2014): 1–154. More recently, Tavormina has edited nine Middle English uroscopical texts, making the texts available for the first time and demonstrating their historical and cultural significance. See Tavormina, ed., *The Dome of Uryne: A Reading Edition of Nine Middle English Uroscopies* (Oxford: EETS, 2019).

6  See Angela Montford, *Health, Sickness, Medicine and the Friars in the Thirteenth and Fourteenth Centuries* (Aldershot: Ashgate, 2004). Faye Marie

Getz also discusses the charity of friar physicians in her detailed analysis of the idea of the medical practitioner in late medieval England. See "The Variety of Medical Practitioners in Medieval England" in *Medicine in the English Middle Ages* (Princeton: Princeton University Press, 1998). For another insightful examination of the role of friar physicians, see Caroline Walker Bynum's discussion of medieval friars' conception of, and relation to, blood in *Wonderful Blood: Theology and Practice in Late Medieval Northern Germany and Beyond* (Philadelphia: University of Pennsylvania Press, 2007) especially chapters 5 (112–32), 7 (153–72) and 8 (173–92).

7 *Liber Uricrisiarum: A Reading Edition*, edited by E. Ruth Harvey, M. Teresa Tavormina, and Sarah Star (Toronto: University of Toronto Press, 2020). I address other partial editions below.

8 Daniel's Latin treatise survives in one manuscript: Glasgow, University Library, Hunterian MS 362. Tavormina discusses the Latin version in her chapter, "The Heirs of Henry Daniel: The Fifteenth- and Sixteenth-Century Legacy of the *Liber Uricrisiarum*," 108–32.

9 See Joanne Jasin, *A Critical Edition of the Middle English "Liber Uricrisiarum" in Wellcome ms. 225 [microform]* (Ann Arbor: University Microfilms International, 1983). Jasin refers to Daniel as a compiler in her later work (see, for example, "The Transmission of Learned Medical Literature in the Middle English *Liber Uricrisiarum*," *Medical History* 37.3 (1993): 14), but she maintains that Daniel's intention in completing the *Liber Uricrisiarum* was to translate the *De urinis* of Isaac Judaeus's "nerhand woord for woord." Jasin's idea has influenced subsequent readers of Daniel. See, for example, Voigts, "Multitudes of Middle English Medicine," 188 and Taavitsainen and Pahta, "Vernacularisation of Scientific and Medical Writing," 13. The latter scholars contend, rightly, that Daniel is a scrupulous editor of his own work; but they, like Jasin, claim that Daniel's thorough editing occurs in spite of his alleged attempt to provide a direct translation of Isaac Judaeus's *De urinis*.

10 See the *Liber Uricrisiarum: A Reading Edition*, 2.2.257, 2.2.306–7, 2.13.393–4, and 3.20.393.

11 See Harvey and Tavormina, "Introduction," *A Reading Edition*, 3–11.

12 For Irma Taavitsainen, Daniel's tendency to include his own "opinion" about some of the information he translates allows him to blur the distinction between "translator" and "commentator." See Taavitsainen, "Transferring Classical Discourse Forms into the Vernacular," *Medical and Scientific Writing in Late Medieval English*, 54. The extent to which Daniel can indeed be considered a commentator exceeds the scope of this project; but, Taavitsainen is undoubtedly correct to observe that Daniel collapses conventional boundaries between, at the very least, "translator" and "commentator."

13  Harvey and Tavormina, "Introduction," *A Reading Edition*, 19.
14  A group of graduate students at the University of Toronto, under the leadership of M. Teresa Tavormina, is currently working towards a critical edition of the herbal. Daniel composed a short treatise on rosemary which was contained within the herbal but also circulated independently. It has been edited by Martti Mäkinen: "Henry Daniel's Rosemary in MS X.90 of the Royal Library, Stockholm," *Neuphilologische Mitteilungen* 103.3: 305–27.
15  London, British Library, Additional MS 27329 and London, British Library, Arundel MS 42.
16  See Jasin, *A Critical Edition of the Middle English "Liber Uricrisiarum" in Wellcome MS 225*, PhD diss., Tulane University, 1983. Despite the title, this is not a critical edition, but rather a transcription and introduction to the text as it is represented London, Wellcome Library, MS 225.
17  See Tom Arvid Johannessen, "The *Liber Uricrisiarum* in Gonville and Caius College, Cambridge, MS 336/725," Master's Thesis, University of Oslo, 2005.
18  See Ralph Hanna, "Henry Daniel's *Liber Uricrisiarum* (Excerpt)," in *Popular and Practical Science of Medieval England*, ed. Lister M. Matheson (East Lansing: Colleagues Press, 1994), 185–218.
19  As Harvey and Tavormina note in their introduction to *A Reading Edition*, we aim with the edition to give scholars access to the text, and hope that a renewed interest in Daniel will lead towards a critical edition sometime in the future. See Harvey and Tavormina, "Introduction," *A Reading Edition*, 30–1.
20  See Harvey and Tavormina, "Introduction," *A Reading Edition*, 20–30.
21  For a detailed account of Langland's revisions and a useful critical bibliography, see Charlotte Brewer, *Editing Piers Plowman: The Evolution of the Text* (Cambridge: Cambridge University Press, 1996).
22  See Sarah Star, "The Textual Worlds of Henry Daniel," *Studies in the Age of Chaucer* 40 (2018): 191–216, cited at 196. Harvey analyses Daniel's audience thoroughly in "Medicine and Science in Chaucer's Day," *The Oxford Handbook of Chaucer*, edited by Suzanne Conklin Akbari and James Simpson (Oxford: Oxford University Press, 2020), 440–55.
23  Star, "Textual Worlds," 203.
24  For more on the textual history of Middle English uroscopies, see Tavormina, "Uroscopy in Middle English."
25  Sarah Star, "Henry Daniel, Medieval English Medicine, and Linguistic Innovation: A Lexicographic Study of Huntington MS HM 505," *Huntington Library Quarterly* 81.1 (2018): 63–106.
26  For more on Daniel's connection to these poets, and to Chaucer in particular, see Star, "Textual Worlds."

# PART ONE

# Contexts

*Chapter One*

## Latin Traditions of Uroscopy

FAITH WALLIS

### Henry Daniel and the Latin Tradition of Uroscopy

Wise Aristotle, as is evident *ex fine primi et principio secundi metha-phisice*, thanks not only those that prior to him put forth or taught wisely in writing, but also those that did not do so wisely, for he found many more subtle things about the matters that others wrote on before. For according to the same Aristotle *in fine 2i libri elenchorum*, the things that are found to have been worked on before by other men are notably extended and increased by those who take them up afterward. And *sequitur*, when something is first discovered, it is wont to increase but little at first, but the increase that follows afterwards is more profitable, *hic ille*. I am not saying this of myself because I am writing new things, but because I am doing it in a new way. I have gathered for those who know how to grasp it in Latin a short treatise containing in full the marrow of this subject, and I wrote it in the tongue that, forsooth, is right dear to me.

In his Latin Prologue to the *Liber Uricrisiarum*,[1] Henry Daniel positions himself as both the heir to a long tradition of Latin writing about uroscopy, and the vanguard of uroscopy's progress. Both claims are conveyed in his implicit comparison of himself to Aristotle, who looked back with a critical eye on the achievements of his predecessors, and then moved forward to surpass them. Though Daniel does not claim to be "writing new things," he does say that he is framing this Latin tradition in a new way, one that is "more profitable" for having synthesised "the marrow of this subject," and then diffused it in English.

Despite Daniel's claim, his Prologue appears in a number of manuscripts not in English, but in Latin. Indeed, an unwary reader, opening the treatise to its first page, might conclude that the *Liber Uricrisiarum* was yet another Latin treatise on urine science. In Cambridge, Gonville and Caius College 180/213, the Prologue ends with Latin verses ("Tu qui eterne manes hunc conservare digneris"), and a Latin explicit paints the author as the expert channel of the Latin uroscopic tradition: "Explicit liber uricrisiarum ex latino in vulgari editus a fr Henrico Daniel ord. pred. omnium scienciarum ac doctrinarum lingue latine yperaspiste et translatore" (Here ends the *Book of the Judgements of Urine* composed out of Latin into the vulgar tongue by Friar Henry Daniel of the Order of Preachers, guardian and translator of all the knowledge and teaching of the Latin language). Indeed, the Latin pedigree of Daniel's learning is flaunted on every page of the *Liber Uricrisiarum*. Latin terminology, glossed in English, is ubiquitous, giving an almost macaronic flavour to his prose. Chapter titles and cross-references are almost always in Latin. Even some commonplace words that one might expect him to simply render in English resolutely retain their Latin forms, words like the names of the seasons or the stages of the human life cycle.[2] Daniel even retains the Latin and Greek names for colours found in his sources, except for "bla" and "whyte."

Daniel's sources were Latin works on medicine and science, and his book's authority depends on reminding the reader of that fact. They include the pillars of the Latin uroscopic tradition – Hippocrates's *Aphorisms*, Theophilus, Isaac Judaeus, Gilles de Corbeil's *Carmen de urinis* and its prose commentary, Gilbert the Englishman's commentary on Gilles, Avicenna's *Canon* – but he also draws on a wide range of works on medical theory (e.g., the *Isagoge* of Joannitius, the *Anatomia Galieni*) and practice (e.g., Constantine the African's *Viaticum*, Johannes de Sancto Paulo's *Breviarium Ypocratis*). This chapter will map the Latin tradition of medical writing dedicated to urine science within which the author of the *Liber Uricrisiarum* situated his own work. At the same time, it will endeavour to explain the uniquely significant role of urine science in Western medicine. The *Liber Uricrisiarum*, after all, is more than a practical guide to uroscopy. In many respects it is a *summa* of anatomy, physiology, and pathology – what medieval authors called the "theory" of medicine. These topics in turn rest upon the physics of the four elements and their interlocking qualities of hot, cold, wet, and dry; consequently, they sweep up cosmology, the seasons and their regimen, and medical astrology. It was the Latin tradition of uroscopic writing that encouraged Daniel to enlarge a treatise on urine into a small encyclopaedia. But it is also the Latin tradition that guided him in turning this knowledge into "judgments," that is, precepts for applying urine science in practice to diagnose the patient's state, and deliver a prognosis.

Four works in particular – Theophilus's *De urinis*, Isaac Judaeus's *De urinis*, Gilles de Corbeil's *Carmen de urinis*, and the *Canon* of

Avicenna – shaped the twofold destiny of urine science as both synony-mous with theory and the cornerstone of practice. These texts extended the boundaries of uroscopy by incorporating anatomical and physio-logical explanations, and by foregrounding the Galenic pathology of fevers, its basis in the humours, and the consequent signs of disorder in the urine. Fevers in turn pointed to the doctrine of critical days, ampli-fied by the translation of Galen's *De crisibus* and already being "astrolo-gized" by the early thirteenth century.[3] Latin urine science, in Laurence Moulinier-Brogi's phrase, became a technique of "reading the whole human being" in the narrow confines of the urine glass or jordan.[4] Urine was the hidden interior processes of the body made visible to the eye, the condensed (and hence obscure) imprint of otherwise ineffable dramas and transformations. Even after it was collected in the jordan, urine might continue to change in sympathy with the alterations un-der way in its native body. Urine's power to signify what was taking place in the living body meant that the study of urines was the study of the workings of life, and of disease itself. This is why urine science became *par excellence* the emblem of the new rational medicine of the central medieval period, and the glass jordan the classic attribute of the learned practitioner. The corollary, however, was that rational uroscopy had to be central to the physician-patient encounter; indeed, patients increasingly regarded it as proof of the competence of the practitioner – his clinical *judgment*. Hence the impulse to theorise urine science and situate it in the broadest possible framework of medical science carried in its wake the need to make that knowledge usable by practitioners.

### The Watershed of the Latin Uroscopy Tradition

The broad stream of Latin literature on urines that flowed past the shores of the *Liber Uricrisiarum* had its headwaters in the Greek medical tradi-tion associated with the name of Hippocrates, and elaborated by Galen. However, a fully articulated theory of how urine is formed, and how its variation signifies internal bodily conditions, only began to take shape in Late Antiquity, and only in Greek texts. During the first millennium of our era, Byzantine Greek and Arabic medical works – commentaries, syntheses of medical science, and specialist works on diagnosis – transformed the scattered references to urine in the classical sources into a fully rationalised semiotics. These Byzantine and Arabic tributaries poured into the Latin stream in the eleventh and twelfth centuries, and changed its course ever after. Latin uroscopy took a theoretical turn.

What this theoretical turn meant can be clarified by looking at the Latin tradition prior to this watershed period.[5] Very few of the Hippocratic treatises or the works of Galen were turned into Latin before 1100, and those that were tended to present urine as a *sign* without a *semiotics*. A good example is Hippocrates's *Aphorisms*, available in Latin with a substantial commentary from the sixth century onwards. Aphorisms 69–83 of *particula* 4 list various morbid appearances of urine and what they indicate. Some of the conditions are problems of the urinary tract itself, such as bladder inflammation (4.77) or rupture of a small renal blood-vessel (4.78). However, other kinds of urine point to more remote pathologies: colourless urine, for example, is an index of brain disease (4.72). A great deal of attention is devoted to urine in fevers. Here urine assumes a prognostic role, announcing a coming crisis: for example, urine exhibiting a "red cloud" on the fourth day of a fever presages a crisis on the seventh day (4.71).[6]

*Aphorisms* does not explain why the colour or the contents of urine signify what they do. This was compensated for in some measure by Hippocrates's *Prognosis*, notably section 12. Here we find a description of baseline healthy urine, and a full suite of parameters for analysing urine according to substance (thick or thin), colour, and precipitates. Healthy urine has a white, smooth, and even deposit of sediment, so if the sediment is pink, but otherwise "healthy," recovery is assured, but will be prolonged. *Prognosis* also introduces the concept of urine as an index of the "ripening" or "digestion" (*pepsis*) and hence resolution of a disease. However, *Prognosis* was only translated into Latin around 1100, so even these elements of a theory of urine long remained unknown in the West.

Galen made major contributions to the science of urines, first by elaborating the anatomy and physiology of urine production as a by-product of the transformation of food into blood,[7] and second, by linking different types of fevers to the four humours, and then correlating these fever-humour combinations to specific changes in urine.[8] Only minute dribbles of this theory found their way into the anonymous Old Latin *Aphorisms* commentary, though. For example, the commentary on *Aphorisms* 4.70 explains that the reason that clear white urine betokens frenzy is that white urine results from excess phlegm, and phlegm in the brain or the vessels leading to the brain causes mental disturbances (a theory reaching back to Hippocrates's *The Sacred Disease*). Unfortunately, this is almost the only place a Latin reader of the first millennium could find even a hint of Galen's larger thinking on the subject of urines.[9]

On the other hand, the early medieval Latin reader was fairly awash in urine lore in the form of catalogues of rules for decoding urines. Many of these works were anonymous or pseudonymous, and open to the kind of creative reorganization, abbreviation, and expansion that was the hallmark of early medieval medical writing.[10] Two examples of this sprawling uroscopy literature will illustrate these points; the *De pulsibus et urinis* variously ascribed to Alexander *medicus* or Galen; and the *Liber medicine orinalibus* of Hermogenas. The first was quite widely diffused; the second is preserved only in MS Montecassino, Biblioteca della Badia 69, 545–50.[11]

Alexander's treatise is organised by disease: the first seven chapters cover fevers, and the remaining twenty-three cover illnesses in roughly head-to-toe order. The style is aphoristic: if X, then Y, X being the type of urine, sometimes combined with an implied diagnosis, and Y the prognosis. The connection of urine to humoral pathology is present, but extremely weak. Alexander deploys the entire range of analytical axes for urine, namely consistency, colour, and contents, but offers no explanation as to why variations occur. Indeed, the ordering of the treatise by disease does not invite systematic description of urine itself. Alexander also used unspecific qualitative terms like "delicate colour" or "cloudy in an evil way," as if the experienced uroscopist would simply know what these meant.

A different approach, but with similar results, is found in the *Liber medicine orinalibus*. Hermogenas's starting point is the urine itself, which can assume one of six possible colours, ranging from white to black. This spectrum is roughly correlated to the dominance of one of the humours over the others, but Hermogenas rarely links the state of urine either to specific disease conditions, or to prognoses. Only the movement of the precipitates in the urine upwards or downwards within the flask is indicative, and only in the most general way. Indeed, any movement seems to signify that the patient or the medication is gaining the upper hand over the disease.[12]

These treatises with named authors are vastly outnumbered by anonymous catalogues of rules for matching urines to diseases or vice versa, but without operating instructions or explanatory background. They breathe the air of divination rather than diagnosis.

## Uroscopy's Theoretical Turn: Theophilus and Isaac Judaeus

A major watershed in the Latin uroscopy tradition is the long twelfth century (ca. 1060–1220), when three very influential texts entered the Latin sphere, one translated from the Greek, another from the Arabic, and the third composed in Latin by a Western European. These were the *De urinis* of Theophilus, the treatise that went by the same Latin title by Isaac Judaeus, i.e., Ishāq ibn Sulaymān al-Isrā'īlī (d. ca. 932–935), and the poem on urines with accompanying prose commentary by Gilles de Corbeil (d. early thirteenth c.).[13]

The precise time and place of the translation of Theophilus's book is unknown, but its early integration into the anthology later called the *Ars medicinae* or *Articella* suggests that, like the other components of this ensemble, it was translated in the region of Salerno or Monte Cassino between 1077 and 1100, and within the patronage network of Archbishop Alfanus of Salerno and Abbot Desiderius of Monte Cassino.[14] These men and their successors were sponsors of the translation activities of Constantine the African (d. ca. 1086–1099), who *inter alia* turned Isaac's medical writings – *De urinis*, *De febribus*, and *Diaetae universales et particulares* – from Arabic into Latin.[15] The two urine treatises are thus closely linked historically. Furthermore, the earliest commentaries on Theophilus drew heavily on Isaac, as well as on other works of Arabic medical science translated by Constantine, particularly the *Pantegni* of Ali ibn al' Abbas al Majūsi (fl. ca. 977). Isaac's treatises were always ascribed properly to him.[16] Theophilus was joined in the new *Articella* ensemble by a fresh translation of Hippocrates's *Aphorisms*, a translation of the *De pulsibus* ascribed in the West to the Byzantine writer Philaretus, and Hippocrates's *Prognosis*. Given the presence of two works on medical semiotics, plus the two works of Hippocrates that most explicitly addressed semiotics, the *Articella* might look like a themed collection of texts on diagnosis and prognosis, were it not for the book that almost invariably heads the anthology. This was the *Isagoge* of "Joannitius," Constantine's translation and adaptation of the *Masā'il fi-tibb* (*Questions about Medicine*) of Hunayn ibn Ishāq (809–887). The *Isagoge* was a digest of Galen's theory of medicine, summarised from his *Art of Medicine* (*Techne iatrike*, or in the West, *Tegni*). The *Isagoge* gave the *Articella* a new identity as a textbook of medical theory. Theophilus's *De urinis* proved to be an ideal vehicle for bringing urine science into this new intellectual setting.[17]

The translation of Theophilus's *De urinis* presented Latin readers for the first time with a coherent explanation of how urine is formed, why it varies in consistency, colour and contents, and how these variations signal physical changes.[18] The underlying models of the body and of disease processes were those of Galen, for which the *Isagoge* now furnished a schematic guide. Like Alexander *medicus*, Theophilus yoked urine science closely to knowledge of fevers; but unlike Alexander, he articulated this connection as one of cause and effect, not just as signifier and signified. The key was the crucial concept of coction. Theophilus represents an important trend in late Antique Greek medical thinking that replaced pulse with urine as the principal focus of semiotic thinking.[19] This new science of urines was based on Galenic humoral pathology, particularly the notion of "coction" or "digestion" as the effect of heat (natural or unnatural) on the humours.[20] Focusing on heat stimulated a more elaborate classification of urine colours. The spectrum from "white" to "black" was theorised as a range from "raw" to "burnt," and the hues between were subdivided into grades of more or less "cooked" that shaded into one another. Terms like *subribicundus* ("reddish") and *subrufus* ("somewhat rufous") go back to classical Latin, but Byzantine uroscopy generated numerous new Greek words, such as *charopos* ("camel-hair"), *inopos* (wine red), and *kyanos* (reddish purple). Thanks to Theophilus, a number of Greek terms were adopted into Latin *tel quel*.[21]

Along with the other components of the *Articella*, Theophilus was the subject of Latin commentaries. The earliest of these, the anonymous suites of *Articella* commentaries called the "Chartres" and "Digby" glosses, were composed in the first quarter of the twelfth century. The first commentary by a named author is ascribed to the famous master Bartholomaeus (fl. ca. 1150–1170).[22] All these commentaries treat *De urinis* to a formal *accessus ad librum*,[23] which gives them an opportunity to define the subject matter and utility of the treatise, as well as the part of philosophy to which it pertains. "Chartres" declares that the usefulness of *De urinis* is "secure knowledge of health, sickness, and the neutral state and their causes" – that is, the threefold division of the subject matter of medicine in Galen's *Tegni*. It pertains to natural philosophy (*physica*) through *theorica*, for "in this science, contemplation alone is exercised."[24] This lofty view of urine science as essentially encompassing the whole art of medicine is echoed by "Digby."[25] Bartholomaeus, however, goes even further, prefacing the *accessus* by situating urine production in the liver, one of the three principal organs governing the entire body identified by Galen's *Tegni*. The workings of the unseen inner parts of the body are known (as Galen asserts) through four signs: swelling, pain, functional damage, and excreta. Urine is the chief example of the last sign. Theophilus's book on urines is to the liver what Philaretus's on pulse is to the heart, thus reinforcing its new identity as a "chapter" in the *Articella* ensemble.[26] In short, *De urinis* is about Galenic physiology and Galenic pathology, and is essentially for teaching medical theory.

Theophilus certainly courts such a reading. He opens his work by situating himself within the history of urine science in terms that anticipate Henry Daniel's. Before him were the great Hippocrates, Galen, and Magnus of Emesa. Hippocrates, however, scattered his references to urine through numerous books, whereas Galen, though a prolific writer, was "inconclusive and obscure" (*indeterminata et obscura*). Magnus discussed types of urines, but omitted prognosis. Hence, Theophilus builds on this heritage, but also improves its usefulness.

Theophilus set the pattern for subsequent urine tracts by starting with a definition of urine and a description of how it is produced that lays special emphasis on how the quality of the urine mirrors the quality of the blood from which it is made, being thin or thick, and of different colours.[27] Healthy natural urine is moderate in consistency (*substantia*), shows a sediment (*hypostasis*) that is white, even and uniform, and is tawny (*ruffa*) or somewhat tawny (*subruffa*) in colour (ch. 3). Urine that is thin in consistency is undigested; thick urine indicates digestion (ch. 4). Theophilus then presents the spectrum of colours of urine (ch. 6) that was destined to become standard in the Latin West. He improves on Hippocrates and Galen by arranging the colours in a systematic gradation from white to black – Aristotle's two primary colours, from which all others are derived by mixture (*De sensu et sensato*).[28]

1 *albus*
2 *lacteus*, or milky-white
3 *glaucus*, like the horny tunic of the eye (light grey)
4 *carapos*, like the hair of a camel
5 *subpallida*, like the decoction of half-raw meat
6 *pallida* [29]
7 *subrufus*, like Celtic gold
8 *rufus*, like pure gold
9 *subrubeus*, like safflower
10 *rubeus*, like true saffron
11 *hyperythros*, "flame" [Angeletti translates "red-purple"]
12 *erythros*, "blood which is pure and unadulterated"
13 *inopos*, like dark wine, or fish sauce [Angeletti translates "vivid-red"]
14 *kianos*, grey (with darker grey = *fuscus*) [Angeletti translates "dark blue"]
15 *cloron*, "like cabbage or grass"
16 violet green
17 emerald green
18 *ysathodes* or woad-green [Angeletti translates "turquoise"]
19 *pelitmon*, "like lead"
20 *niger*

Then follow various combinations of consistencies (thin, thick, and middling) with these colours, progressing from light to dark (chs. 7–8).

Colours lighter than *subruffa/ruffa* signify insufficient digestion, due to weakness of natural heat or excessive phlegm. As the colours approach *subruffa* the urine becomes a more positive sign, and the dominant humour shifts to blood. Finally, thick black urine betokens melancholy or scorching of blood.

Now Theophilus turns to precipitates (ch. 10–11): sediment lying on the bottom of the urine (*hypostasis*), suspended matter in the middle (*eneorima*), and surface nebulosities (*nubes*) (chs. 12–14). Finally, Theophilus considers special diagnostic signs, namely: oily urine (indicating the "melting" of kidney fat); fragmented precipitates indicating dissolution of the flesh from excessive heat ("husk-like" [*petaloides*], "bran-like" [*furfuree*], and "mealy" [*crinoides*]); and bad smell, indicating putrefaction of the humours. The treatise closes by correlating consistency of the liquid part of urine to consistency of the precipitate.

Here at last is a mature science of urine, fully articulated with respect to the physics of the four qualities, explained in relation to the anatomy and physiology of nutrition, and rationally aligned to a typology of fevers. Theophilus could be fully cross-referenced to the summary of Galenic doctrine found in the *Isagoge* of Joannitius; conversely, he supplied a missing key to the Hippocratic *Aphorisms* and *Prognosis*.

The earliest commentaries on Theophilus, however, could only make sense of the work by drawing on another account, the *De urinis* of Isaac Judaeus, as rendered into Latin by Constantine the African. The Constantinian corpus of Arabic-Latin translations and the *Articella* are closely intertwined not only in their mutual influence, but in their transmission. Isaac's *De urinis* could circulate as part of a larger Constantine ensemble, or as one component of an "Isaac Corpus" along with *Dietae uniuersales et particulares* and *De febribus* (e.g., Durham, Cathedral Library C.IV.13, Philadelphia, University of Pennsylvania Library Schoenberg 24). *De urinis* might accompany the *Articella* (e.g., in Erfurt, Wissenschaftliche Bibliothek Amplon. F. 286, London BL Harley 3140), but it could also be aggregated with other texts on urines (e.g., with Maurus of Salerno[30] in Paris BNF lat. 10237; with Gilles de Corbeil in Cambridge, Corpus Christi College 551). Though never a formal part of any university medical curriculum,[31] Isaac's treatise on urine remained a standard work. Bartholomaeus's commentary on Theophilus not only cites passages from Isaac Judaeus's *De urinis*, but also recognises that Isaac provides perspectives and information missing in the Byzantine treatise. For example, commenting on Theophilus's definition of healthy urine (ch. 3), Bartholomaeus begins by observing that Isaac's book contains instructions for how to collect urine and carry out the inspection – matters not treated by Theophilus. "Therefore let us speak about this, lest it not be covered anywhere (Dicamus igitur nos idem, ne nusquam dicatur)."[32] Hence Isaac's *De urinis* cemented the relationship of uroscopy to the body of theory that underpinned the new approach to medicine.

What made Isaac's *De urinis* so valuable? Apart from the advice on collecting and inspecting urine, Isaac's treatise covers much of the same ground as Theophilus's. However, *De urinis* supplied more of what medicine's theoretical turn demanded than Theophilus did. For example, Isaac's opening chapter on the nature of urine maps the production of urine and its liquid and solid components across the three-stage model of digestion destined to become standard through Avicenna, *Canon* Book 1, Fen 1, doctrina 4, ch. 2, and which is featured in Book 1, ch. 3 of the *Liber Uricrisiarum*. Isaac also cemented the relationship of urine to fever pathology by showing how residues not expelled in urine could cause illness. Indeed, Isaac's own *De febribus* was often read as the complement of his *De urinis*. Isaac's pathology was also more sophisticated than Theophilus's. A comparison here between the treatment of oily urine in the two texts is illuminating, not least because Henry Daniel silently incorporated Isaac's interpretation (*Liber Uricrisiarum* 3.8). Theophilus regards oily urine as a sign of kidney disease involving the melting of the fat around the kidneys. Fat that appears in the urine comes directly from the kidneys, since the kidneys are close to the urinary tract. Fat deposited elsewhere in the body is too remote, even when dissolved, to appear in the urine. Isaac, on the other hand, nuances this explanation by factoring in the presence or absence of fever. If there is no fever, and the fat appears immediately upon urination, floating on top of the urine, the problem indeed lies in the kidneys. But if there is a continuous fever, one should suspect consumption of the whole body, the heat of the fever "melting" even remote body fat. Hence an additional test should be applied: whether the urine is "decocted" or "raw." Urine that signifies melting of kidney fat is "decocted," but "raw" urine shows that the body as a whole is not able to decoct the urine properly because it is labouring under grievous disease, one that causes wasting, and the appearance of oil in the urine.[33]

The intellectual advantages of Isaac's treatise were offset by some practical problems. His discussion of oily urine, for instance, is buried in the chapter on urine colours. While Theophilus plods methodically along a chromatic spectrum from white to black, Isaac starts with the four primary colours associated with the four humours: *citrinissimus* (choler), *rubeus* (blood), white (phlegm), and *nigerissimus* (melancholy). The actual colour of urine depends on whether one humour dominates, with another humour present in a smaller quantity, or whether a pair of humours exerts a combined influence. Thus instead of moving step-wise along a spectrum from white to black, Isaac orders his exposition from simple to compound. In the first case, the following colours result: *citrinus* (composed of *citrinissimus* and white, i.e., phlegm plus some red bile), *igneus* (*rubeus* and *citrinus*, i.e., blood plus some red bile), *purpureus* (*nigerrimus* and red, i.e., blood tending towards melancholy) and *cinericius* (black and white. i.e., phlegm and melancholy). Then he fills in the gaps in the spectrum with the shades produced by combinations of two humours. For example, between *albus* and *citrinus* are egg-yolk (*quasi uitellum*) and bright yellow (*clara citrinitas*), depending on the rel-ative strength of red bile and phlegm. This is undoubtedly one reason why Isaac's typology of urine colours was not broadly adopted. Henry Daniel follows Theophilus's scheme, though Isaac's influence is visi-ble in the fact that Daniel's spectrum starts with black-*liuidus*-white. In sum, the richness and subtlety of Isaac's text may actually have made it less attractive for teaching, and less easy to translate into memorable clinical guidelines.

### Gilles de Corbeil and His Commentators: Urine Science Made Operational

The tension between packaging urine science as medical theory, and packaging urine science for practice, was resolved by the most success-ful work of this genre composed in the Middle Ages, the *Carmen de urinis* of Gilles de Corbeil (d. ca. 1224)[34] and its prose commentary. This commentary is possibly from the pen of Gilles himself; but even if it is not, it was such a precocious and consistent companion to the poem that the two works should be treated as one.

In some ways the poem seems a regression. It is based on Theophi-lus, but condenses *De urinis* by omitting the theory and reframing the contents as *regulae* or guidelines for matching urine type to disease. The language is terse and aphoristic, easy to memorise but devoid of expla-nation. Though he claims in the prologue to follow *antiquorum scriptis*, Gilles cites no sources, though his epilogue pays homage to the teach-ing of his Salernitan masters Petrus Musandinus, Salernus, Urso, and Maurus.[35] In another respect, though, the *Carmen* represented a signif-icant advance. It was the first work to package the new Greco-Arabic urine science in a form that could be readily taught to, and used by, practitioners. Indeed, Mireille Ausécache argues that Gilles intended all of his medical works (*De urinis, De pulsibus, De uirtutibus et laudibus compositorum medicaminum*) to supplement the *Articella* by providing applications of its teaching that were suitable for practice.[36]

The poem's real value emerges when it is placed alongside its prose "Standard Commentary."[37] This text unpacked the gnomic phrases of the poem, and provided the missing scientific background in precisely the terms demanded by scholastic academic practice. An example will illustrate this. The verse *Carmina* introduces Theophilus's twenty colours of urine without any explanation:

Bis deni urinam possunt variare colores
Quos ex subscriptis poteris perpendere formis.[38]

(Twenty are the possible colours of urine
Which you can learn from what is described below.)

The Commentary fills in the background:

In this chapter he shows how many colours of urine there are. There are twenty, and there are a number of ways of distinguishing these colours. Colours are distinguished according to quality, according to the nature of decoction and digestion, and thirdly, according to the properties of the humours. This distinction is made according to properties: some are more intense, some less intense, and others in between. All below "yellowish" (*subcitrinus*) are less intense, all above "rufous" are said to be more intense. In between are yellow (*citrinus*), yellowish, rufous, and somewhat rufous. This distinction of colour applies to natural coction. Some signify mortification (like black, livid); others, lack of digestion (like white, milky, glaucus and tawny); some incipient but incomplete digestion (like pallid, somewhat pallid, and yellowish bordering on pallid); and a fourth <category indicates> complete digestion (yellow, somewhat rufous, rufus). A fifth <indicates> excessive digestion (*inops* [purple-red] and *kianos* [grey]), and a seventh, excessive scorching and death (green, black). But an objection can be raised: why do we begin <the series> and end it with black? We should respond by making this distinction: because one <black> is the colour caused by mortification due to cold and the extinction of heat, while the other one is caused by extreme scorching. Thus the diversity of effect is to be distinguished according to the different cause. The distinction according to humours is straightforward. For some colours signify red bile, others phlegm, others melancholy, and others blood. But to signify the humours, one should add their combination with consistencies.[39]

The Commentary has thus deftly fused Theophilus's thermal model with Isaac's humoral schema of urine colours.

Theophilus, Isaac, Galen, Hippocrates, and Salernitan masters like Johannes de Sancto Paulo are liberally quoted in the Commentary, which also, it should be noted, introduces *quaestiones*. Though it was not officially part of a university medical curriculum, the Commentary indicates that the *Carmen* was undoubtedly read and studied in academic milieux. The combination of the mnemonic poem and the scholastic prose gloss was so successful that it inspired a number of prominent medical writers and teachers to improve on the formula. Though the commentary on Gilles ascribed to Gentile da Foligno ("Ingenii uires. Auctor more recto scribendo ...") appeared in the printed edition of Padua (1483: GW 00268) and Venice (1494/95), Gilbert the Englishman's gloss, composed in the middle of the thirteenth century, was at least as popular, surviving in a dozen manuscripts.[40] Gilbert enhanced the Standard Commentary with a stronger admixture of Aristotle and, above all, Avicenna and Averroes.[41]

## Avicenna

The exposition of urine in Avicenna's *Canon* (Book 1, fen 2, doct. 3) took on extraordinary importance as the authority of this work grew to dominate university medicine all across Western Europe.[42] Taddeo Alderotti of Bologna and his students, particularly Gentile da Foligno, were the first to compose detailed commentaries on this text in Latin, and they were followed by Parisian masters like Jacques Despars.[43] It was the seamless unity of the *Canon* and its analytical character that was most compelling to medieval readers.

The urine chapters are embedded in the third *doctrina* of *fen* 2 of Book 1, devoted to "signs" – one of Galen's three divisions of theory, namely body, signs, and causes (of disease). The treatment of urines in *fen* 2, *doctrina* 3, therefore, concentrated exclusively on urine as sign. That being said, it was semiotics on a highly analytical register. Where other treatises aimed to catalogue all possible combinations of colour and consistency, or colour and precipitates, Avicenna concentrates on how each dimension carries significance. It therefore indicates general processes and trends, and only rarely particular diagnoses. For example, the chapter on the colours of urine associates four key colours with the four humours, and the shades with different intensities of the humour. Not only is Avicenna's vocabulary of colours difficult to align with the (by now) standard spectrum of Theophilus and Gilles, but his subtle analysis is oriented to scientific reasoning rather than clinical application. Concerning red urine, for example:

> ... shades of redness [*rubedinis*] such as rosy [*roseus*], dark red [*rubeus obscurus*] and dusty red [*rubeus puluerulentus*] all signify the dominance of blood. And all that are of a colour bordering on saffron [*zahafarano*] signify the dominance of red bile. And when it approaches a powdery <colour>

it signifies the dominance of blood. ... If these display a certain thin consistency, it signifies a trend towards maturation has already begun, even
if this does not appear in the sample in hand. If citrinity becomes stronger
and comes to the point of fieryness [*igneitatis ... terminum*] is shows that
heat is relentlessly advancing ... And if brightness [*claritas*] increases, heat
is already starting to diminish.[44]

Consequently, Avicenna was not heavily exploited by commentators
on Gilles such as Gilbertus Anglicus; even Bernard of Gordon's *De
urinis* makes only incidental references to Avicenna, often to indicate
his agreement or disagreement with Galen (e.g., ch. 20), or with Theophilus and Isaac (ch. 24).[45] Even the chapter of the smell of urine (25)
does not draw on Avicenna's chapter on the same topic. It is thus all
the more interesting to find Henry Daniel drawing on the *Canon*. While
these references are not abundant, neither do they seem to be at second
hand. This testifies to Daniel's medical learning, and his diligence in
seeking out all that Latin urine science could contribute to his project.

## Conclusion

This overview of Latin urine science highlights a number of characteristic features of the tradition. First, its long early medieval history as catalogues of *regulae* and *signa* was never entirely eclipsed by the theoretical
turn of the twelfth century. Indeed, the success of Gilles de Corbeil's
work lay precisely in restoring the clinical usability of urine science in
the *Carmen*, while retaining its theoretical support in the form of the
prose commentary. Urine science became, particularly in the Salernitan
period, an ideal framework for bridging Galenic theory and the needs
of diagnosis as a critical preparation for therapeutic intervention. Diagnosis in many respects *was* practice, particularly for theory-minded
clinicians, and urine (like pulse) was gratifyingly susceptible to analysis along rational axes, notably the colour spectrum. This gave urine an
abstract and universal character.

A second feature is the priority of the translation of Theophilus's *De
urinis*, which created a Latin terminology for colours and precipitates
that resisted the influence of more sophisticated works, such as Isaac
Judaeus's *De urinis* and the *Canon* of Avicenna. The triumph of this
lexicon was assured by Gilles de Corbeil, and accepted with only minor adjustments by Bernard of Gordon, and by Henry Daniel himself.
That being said, Henry Daniel's *Liber Uricrisiarum* stands out from the
Latin tradition in a number of ways. It is not a commentary on Theophilus or Gilles, but an autonomous treatise. There were not many such

composed in Latin in the later medieval period, apart from Bernard of Gordon's, and there were certainly not many of the length and detail of the *Liber Uricrisiarum*. Daniel's book also departs from Latin models in its encyclopaedic scope, for he uses urine as an anchor or matrix for assembling a sweeping range of medical and scientific information, from signs of pregnancy to finding the position of the moon in the zodiac. While his raw materials were the staples of Latin uroscopy, Henry Daniel's final confection was original, and entirely his own.

NOTES

1   The Latin Prologue appears in Cambridge University Library MS Ff.2.6, ff. 1r–v, Cambridge Gonville and Caius College MS 180/213 f. 1r, Oxford Bodleian Library MS Ashmole 1404 ff. 3r–4r, and San Marino, Huntington Library 505, ff. 1r–v. The translation is mine. The phrase "in Latin" in the final sentence does not appear in the Ashmole and Gonville and Caius (though it does in the Cambridge University Library and Huntington copies), and in fact is difficult to make sense of, as those who "know how to grasp it" (capere sciunt / for þam þat kan take it) in Latin do not need a translation.

2   See *Liber Uricrisiarum: A Reading Edition*, edited by E. Ruth Harvey, M. Teresa Tavormina, and Sarah Star (University of Toronto Press, 2020), 1.4.387–404.

3   Cornelius O'Boyle, *Medieval Prognosis and Astrology. A Working Edition of the Aggregationes de crisi et creticis diebus: with Introduction and English Summary* (Cambridge: Wellcome Unit for the History of Medicine, 1991); Laurence Moulinier-Brogi, *Guillaume l'Anglais, le frondeur de l'uroscopie médiévale (XIIIe siècle)* (Geneva: Droz, 2011). Henry Daniel does not develop a fully astrologised uroscopy like William the Englishman's, but he does insert in Book 2 an extended digression on astronomy and astrology. Here, the only hint of a link to uroscopy is the conventional zodiacal melothesia (the schema matching signs of the zodiac to zones of the human body), and the inclusion of the four humours among the qualities attached to different planets and zodiac signs. The digression is somewhat improbably triggered by a reference to "wandering fevers," so its inclusion may indicate that Daniel had a stronger interest in astro-uroscopy than he revealed.

4   Laurence Moulinier-Brogi, *L'Uroscopie au Moyen Âge. "Lire dans un verre la nature de l'homme"* (Paris: Honoré Champion, 2012).

5   On ancient urine science, see Valentina Gazzaniga, "Urology and Uroscopy from Hippocrates to Roman Medicine," in Luciana Rita Angeletti,

Berenice Cabarro, and Valentina Gazzaniga, eds. *Il De urinis di Teofilo Protospatario: centralità di un segno clinico.* Medicina nei secoli, n.s. suppl. (Rome: Casa editrice Università La Sapienza, 2009), 175–89.

6   Gazzaniga, "Urology and Uroscopy" (2009), 180–1.

7   Ibid., 175–9.

8   The principal texts are: *On natural faculties, On crises* and Book 2 of *Therapeutics to Glaucon*: see D.W. Peterson, "Galen's 'Therapeutics to Glaucon' and its Early Commentaries," PhD diss., Johns Hopkins University, 1974, ch. 3, esp. p. 97. A summary of the urine doctrine in Galen's *De crisibus* was transmitted via Oribasius's *Synopsis* 6.4: *Oeuvres d'Oribase*, ed. U.C. Bussemaker, Charles Daremberg and Auguste Molinier, 6 vols. (Paris: 1873–1876), vol. 6, pp. 97–8.

9   Faith Wallis, "Signs and Senses: Diagnosis and Prognosis in Early Medieval Pulse and Urine Texts," *Social History of Medicine* 13.2 (2000): 265–78, at 275. Some fragments of theory are found in Caelius Aurelanus, Celsus and others: see Faith Wallis, "Inventing Diagnosis: Theophilus's *De urinis* in the Classroom," *Dynamis* 20 (2000): 31–73, at 36.

10  Faith Wallis, "The Experience of the Book: Manuscripts, Texts, and the Role of Epistemology in Early Medieval Medicine," in *Knowledge and the Scholarly Medical Traditions*, ed. Don G. Bates (Cambridge: Cambridge University Press, 1995), 101–26. The indispensable guide to this phenomenon in relation to early medieval uroscopy (particularly the ps-Galen *De urinis*) remains Gundolf Keil, *Die urognostische Praxis in Vor- und Frühsalernitanischer Zeit* (Habilitationsschrift, Albert-Ludwigs-Universität, Freiburg im Breisgau, 1970).

11  Both works are discussed in detail in Wallis, "Signs and Senses," 265–78. The critical edition is by M. Stoffregen, "Eine frühmittelalterliche lateinische Übersetzung des byzantinischen Puls- und Urintraktats des Alexandros," PhD diss., Freie Universität Berlin, 1977.

12  Luigi Iorio and Faustino Avagliano, "Observations on the *Liber medicine orinalibus* by Hermogenes," *American Journal of Nephrology* 19, 2 (1999): 185–8, with English translation of the text. There is no critical edition of the Latin original.

13  Laurence Moulinier-Brogi, "La science des urines de Maurus de Salerne et les *Sinthomata Magistri Mauri* inédits," in *La Scuola medica Salernitana. Gli autori et I testi*, ed. Danielle Jacquart and Agostino Paravicini Bagliani (Florence: SISMEL/Edizioni del Galluzzo, 2007), 263.

14  See Wallis, "Inventing Diagnosis," 31–73; Giles Gasper and Faith Wallis, "Anselm and the *Articella*," *Traditio* 59 (2004): 129–74; Faith Wallis, "Why was the Aphorisms of Hippocrates Re-Translated in the Eleventh Century?" In *Vehicles of Transmission, Translation and Transformation*, ed. Carlos Fraenkel, Jamie Fumo, Faith Wallis and Robert Wisnovsky (Turnhout: Brepols, 2011), 179–99.

15  On Isaac, see Danielle Jacquart and Françoise Micheau, *La médecine arabe et l'occident médiéval*. (Paris: Maisonneuve & Larose, 1990), 113–15; Danielle Jacquart, "La place d'Isaac Israeili dans la médicine médiévale," *Veslius* special number (1998): 19–27; and the magisterial study of *De febribus* by Raphaela Veit, *Das Buch der Fieber des Isaac Israeli und seine Bedeutung im lateinischen Westen: ein Beitrag zur Rezeption arabischer Wissenschaft im Abendland*, Sudhoffs Archiv Beiheft 51 (Stuttgart: Franz Steiner 2003).

16  A medieval legend about Constantine claims that he was inspired to translate Arabic medical works precisely because the "Latins" had no uroscopic theory: ed. R. Creutz, "Die Ehrenrettung Konstantins von Afrika," *Studien und Mitteilungen des Benediktiner Ordens* 49 (1931): 40–1; trans. Faith Wallis, *Medieval Medicine: A Reader* pp. 138–9. Another translation by Francis Newton is printed in *Mediterranean Passages: Readings from Dido to Derrida*, ed. Miriam Cooke, Erdağ Göknar, and Grant Parker (Chapel Hill: University of North Carolina Press, 2008), 116–17. See also Charles Burnett, "The Legend of Constantine the African," in *The Medieval Legends of Philosophers and Scholars* = Micrologus 21 (Florence: SISMEL/Edizione del Galluzzo, 2013), 277–94, and Raphaela Veit, "Quellenkundliches zu Leben und Werk von Constantinus Africanus," *Deutsches Archiv für Erforschung des Mittelalters* 59 (2003): 121–52.

17  This process is discussed by Luciana Rita Angeletti and Valentina Gazzaniga, "Theophilus' *Auctoritas*: The Role of *De urinis* in the Medical Curriculum of the 12th and 13th Centuries," *American Journal of Nephrology* 19 (1999): 165–71, and by Faith Wallis, "Inventing Diagnosis."

18  The Latin text of Theophilus has been critically edited by Sonya Dase, *Liber urinarum a uoce Theophili. Edition einer Übersetzung des 12. Jahrhunderts mit ausführlichem Glossar*. Marburg: Tectum Verlag, 1999. This is the printed version of her 1997 Osnabruck doctoral dissertation. The text has been translated into Italian and English by Luciana Rita Angeletti, Berenice Cavarra, and Valentina Gazzaniga, in *Il De urinis di Teofilo Protospatario* pp. 101–24 (Italian) and 255–74 (English). The Greek text was edited by Julius Ludwig Ideler, *Physici et medici Graeci minores* vol. 1 (Berlin: Reimer, 1841; rpt. Amsterdam: Adolf M. Hakkert, 1963 and Angeletti, Cavarra and Gazzaniga, 139–62). On controversies concerning the identity and dates of Theophilus (which range from the seventh to the ninth centuries), see Berenice Cavarra, "The *De urinis* of Theophilus," in *Il De urinis di Teofilo Protospatario*, 217–23.

19  On Late Antique and early Byzantine urine science in general, see Berenice Cavarra, "Medicine and Uroscopy, from IVth Cent. BC to VII AD," in *Il De urinis di Teofilo Protospatario*, 191–216; K. Dimitriadis, *Byzantinische Uroskopie*. (PhD diss., Bonn, 1971), esp. pp. 45–55 on Theophilus.

20  Moulinier-Brogi, *L'Uroscopie*, 45, 60; and "La science des urines," 263.

21  Moulinier-Brogi, *L'Uroscopie*, 153–4. On Theophilus's colour terminology, see P.G. Maxwell-Stuart, *Studies in Greek Colour Terminology* (Leiden: Brill, 1981).

22  Wallis, "Inventing Diagnosis," 41–8; Wallis, "The *Articella* Commentaries of Magister Bartholomaeus," in *La Scuola medica salernitana: gli autori e i testi*, ed. Danielle Jacquart and Agostino Paravicini Bagliani (Florence: SISMEL/Edizioni, 2007), 125–64.

23  Wallis, "Inventing Diagnosis," 48–52.

24  London, BL Royal 8.C.IV f. 163r: "Vtilitas uero est firma cognitio sanitatis. egritudinis. et neutralitatis. cum causis eorum. physice supponitur tantum per teoricam. In hac enim scientia sola contemplatio operatur."

25  Oxford, Bodleian Library Digby 108, ff. 76r–v: "Vtilitas est maxima scilicet significationis urine in sanis egris et neutris perfecta noticia. Physice hunc libellum supponi nemo dubitat cum de rerum contemplationibus agat."

26  Winchester, Winchester College Library MS 24, f. 157va: "Omnium membrorum uita et nutrimentum a corde et epate procedit. A corde uita, unde et in Pantegni spiritualis uirtus uiuificans appellatur et spiritus qui a corde procedit uitalis dicitur quo membra calent actu et uiuificantur. Ab epate uero sanguinem ad nutrimentum memborum omnium procedere nemo dubitat. Vnde et quemadmodum apud Galienum in Tegni habetur, horum membrorum principalium complexionem totum corpus sequitur. Cuiuscumque enim complexionis cor fuerit eiusdem et totum corpus erit nisi epar contra operetur et cuiuscumque epar eiusdem et totum corpus nisi cor contra operetur. Ideoque et signa quibus de epate et corde certificamur plurimum ad noticiam tocius corporis ualent. Cum autem membrorum non apparentium IIIIor modis cognitiones habe<a>ntur id est per tumores et dolores per operationum lesiones per egestiones, ut Galienus in Tegni testatur, per pulsum et per urinam de corde et epate plurimum certificamur, cordis per pulsum epatis per urinam noticiam habentes. Ideoque auctores de hiis duobus discretum tractatum instituere ut Philaretus de pulsu, Theophilus uero deinde librum istum edidit in cuius principio hec sunt attendenda." (The life and nutriment of all parts of the body proceeds from the heart and from the liver. From the heart, life: hence in the *Pantegni* the spiritual virtue is called "life-giving" and the spirit which proceeds from the heart, by whose action the parts of the body are warmed and vivified is called "vital." No one doubts that the blood and nutriment of all the parts <of the body> proceed from the liver. Hence as Galen opines in the *Tegni*, the whole body follows the complexion of the principal body parts [i.e., *liver, heart, brain and testicles*]. So whatever the complexion of the heart is, that will be the complexion of the entire body unless the liver countervails, and whatever the complexion of the liver is, will be the complexion of the entire body unless the heart countervails.

In consequence the signs by which we ascertain <the complexion of> the liver and the heart are largely valid for gathering information about the entire body. As knowledge of the inconspicuous parts <of the body> is obtained in four ways, namely by swelling, pain, defective function, and evacuations, as Galen attests in the *Tegni*, through the pulse and the urine we ascertain for the most part <the condition of> the heart and the liver, gaining information about the heart from the pulse and about the liver from the urine. Therefore the authorities established separate treatises for these two, as Philaretus on the pulse, and Theophilus likewise. Hence he composed this book, at the outset of which the following matters must be considered.) This is the version of Bartholomaeus's commentary designated the "main" recension by Paul Oskar Kristeller, "Bartholomaeus, Musandinus and Maurus of Salerno and other Early Commentators of the Articella, with a Tentative List of Texts and Manuscripts." *Italia medioevale e umanistica* 29 (1976): 57–87; translated, with additions and corrections, as "Bartolomeo, Musandino, Mauro di Salerno e altri antichi commentatori dell'*Articella*, con un elenco di testi e di manoscritti," in *Studi sulla scuola medica salernitana* (Naples: Istituto italiano per gli studi filosofici, 1986), 97–151. Kristeller's "variant" version, which survives in as many manuscripts as the "main" one, begins with Galen's four indicators, and expands on the different kinds of *egestiones* in relation to Galenic *virtutes* and *operationes*: see MS Erfurt, Wissenschaftliche Bibliothek, Amplon. Q 175, f. 58va–b.

27  Theophilus's text is summarised by Luciana R. Angeletti, "Textual Examination," in *Il De urinis di Teofilo Protospatario*, 225–53. A detailed discussion of the "filtrate" theory is presented by Luciana Rita Angeletti and Bernice Cavarra, "Critical and Historical Approach to Theophilus's *De urinis*. Urine as Blood's Percolation made by the Kidney and Uroscopy in the Middle Ages." *American Journal of Nephrology* 14 (1994): 282–9.

28  Angeletti, "Textual examination," 238–40.

29  Two further shades of yellow, *ypoxanthos* and *xanthos*, while not included in the chapter on urine colours, are mentioned in Theophilus's discussion in chs. 7–8 of combinations of colours with consistencies.

30  Maurus (d. ca. 1214) was a famous teacher in Salerno, and composed *inter alia* two innovative works on urines: *Regulae urinarum* and *Sinthomata Magistri Mauri*. He was admired by Gilles de Corbeil: Laurence Moulinier, "La science des urines." On Maurus and other Salernitan writers on urine science, notably Urso of Calabria, see Massimo Oldoni, "Uroscopy in the Salerno School of Medicine," *American Journal of Nephrology* 14 (1994): 483–7.

31  Moulinier, *L'Uroscopie* p. 67, n. 248 and Jacquart and Micheau both cite the 1270–1274 curriculum of the medical faculty of Paris, but the text of the

statute only mentions "the *Viaticum* and *other works* by Isaac": H. Denifle and E. Chatelain, *Cartularium Universitatis Parisiensis* (Paris: Delalaine, 1889–1897), vol. 1, 516–17. The statutes of Montpellier and Bologna prescribe some of Isaac's works, but not *De urinis*: Jacquart and Micheau 181, 192. Petrus Hispanus's commentary accompanies all of Isaac's works in the Lyon 1515 *Omnia opera Ysaac* including *De urinis* on ff. 156ra–203rb. Four other commentaries are listed in Thorndike and Kibre's *Incipits of Medieval Scientific Works in Latin* (Cambridge MA: Mediaeval Academy of America, 1963), cols. 239, 397, 781, 614; all but one are anonymous, and all survive in only a single manuscript.

32  Erfurt, Wissenschaftliche Bibliothek Amplon. Q 125 f. 59va. Henry Daniel reproduces Isaac's advice in Book 1, ch. 6 of the *Liber Uricrisiarum*.

33  Isaac Judaeus, *De urinis* 5, *Omnia opera Ysaac* (Lyon, 1515), vol. 1, f. 175rb: "Secundus modus significans dissolui pinguedinem in renibus: liquor est coctus et digestus uirtutem membrorum demonstrans: quia nondum ad ea passiones perueniunt. Significans consumptionem corporis liquor est crudus et indigestus: quia membra defecta sunt in decoctione urine propter passiones eorum: et inceptam consumptionem ipsorum." Isaac's treatise was transcribed from this edition, and allegedly collated with Leipzig Universitätsbibliothek 1154 (but without critical apparatus), in the 1919 Leipzig MD thesis by Johannes Peine, "Die Harnschrift des Isaac Judaeus."

34  On Gilles's life and work, see Mireille Ausécache's introduction to her edition of Gilles's *Liber de uirtutibus et laudibus compositorum medicaminum* (Florence: SISMEL/Edizioni del Galluzzo, 2017), esp. 11–15, and Mireille Ausécache, "Gilles de Corbeil ou le médecin pédagogique au tournant des XIIe et XIIIe siècles," *Early Science and Medicine* 3 (1998): 187–215. Ausécache's work supplants C. Vieillard, *Essai sur la société médicale et religieuse au XIIe siècle: Gilles de Corbeil. ...* Paris: Honoré Champion, 1909.

35  Ausécache, *Liber de uirtutibus*, 61–2.

36  Ausécache, *Liber de uirtutibus*, 19.

37  This and other commentaries on the *Carmen de urinis* were first surveyed by Karl Sudhoff, "Commentatoren der Harnverse des Gilles de Corbeil," *Archeion* 11 (1929): 128–35. Sudhoff ascribed the Standard Commentary to Gilles himself (pp. 132) on the basis of some medieval rubrics. The Standard Commentary begins "Liber iste ..." or "Iste liber ..." or "Liber quem proponimus legendum ...": the list of manuscripts enumerated in Thorndike and Kibre's *Catalogue of Incipits* (cols. 788–91, 821) is far from complete; Sudhoff (131) adds Leipzig Universitätsbibliothek 1176 and 1215, and Erfurt, Amplon F 176 and Q 178.

38  Ed. Ludwig Choulant, *Aegidii Corboliensis carmina medica* (Leipzig: J.B. Hirschfeld, 1826), p. 5, lines 19–20. Choulant's edition was reprinted, with

accompanying French translation, in C. Vieillard, *L'Urologie et les médecins urologues dans la médecine ancienne* (Paris: F.R. de Rudeval, 1903), 267–301.

39  Latin text in London, British Library Sloane MS 282, ff. 20v–21r; transcription by E. Ruth Harvey. The translation is mine.

40  *Inc.* Sicut dicit Constantinus in Pantegni … To the manuscripts listed in Thorndike and Kibre (1483), should be added London, Wellcome Library 547, Oxford, New College 170, Leipzig Universitätsbibliothek 1172 and 1174, and Vienna Nationalbibliothek 2310 (cf. Sudhoff, "Commentatoren," 133).

41  To Michael McVaugh, this is persuasive evidence that Gilbert was educated, and perhaps taught, in Paris: "Who was Gilbert the Englishman?" in *The Study of Medieval Manuscripts in England: Festschrift in Honor of Richard W. Pfaff* ed. George Hardin Brown and Linda Ehrsam Voigts (Tempe: Arizona Center for Medieval and Renaissance Studies in collaboration with Brepols, 2010), 302–4.

42  Danielle Jacquart, "La réception du Canon d'Avicenne: comparaison entre Montpellier et Paris au XIIIe et XIVe siècles," in *Histoire de l'École médicale de Montpellier. Actes du 110e Congrès national des Sociétés savantes (Montpellier 1985)* (Paris: C.T.H.S., 1985), v. 2, 68–77; Joël Chandelier, *Avicenne et la médecine en Italie: le Canon dans les universités (1200–1350)* (Paris: Champion 2017); Nancy Siraisi, *Avicenna in Renaissance Italy: The Canon and Medical teaching in Italian Universities after 1500* (Princeton: Princeton University Press, 1987).

43  On Taddeo and his school, see Nancy Siraisi, *Taddeo Alderotti and his Pupils: Two Generations of Italian Medical Learning* (Princeton: Princeton University Press, 1981). On Gentile, see Roger French, *Canonical Medicine: Gentile da Foligno and Scholasticism* (Leiden: Brill, 2001). On Despars, Danielle Jacquart, "Le regard d'un médecin sur son temps: Jacques Despars (1380?–1458)," *Bibliothèque de l'École des chartes* 138 (1980): 35–86.

44  … gradus rubedinis sicut roseus et rubeus obscurus: et rubeus puluerulentus et omnes quod sanguinis dominium significant. Et in omnibus in quibus est color zahafarano attinens est significatio dominii colere rubee. Et in omnibus que puluerulento attinent est significatio dominii sanguinis. … Quod si ibi fuerit tenuitas aliquam maturationis significat dispositionem et quod iam incepit et si non appareat in subjecta. Si autem citrinitas fortior fiat et usque ad igneitatis perueniat terminum et ad finem in ea significat quod calor incessanter processit. *Canon* Book 1, fen 2 doct. 3, sum. 2, c. 2 (Lyon: Symphorien Champier, 1522), f. 40vb.

45  *De urinis*, in *Bernardi Gordonii opus, Lilium medicinae inscriptum … Vni cum aliquot aliis eius libellis* (Lyon, Guliel. Rouillius, 1574), 728–824.

## Chapter Two

ℰᴗ

# Translation, Comparison, and Adaptation: Latin Verse Herbals in the *Aaron Danielis*

WINSTON BLACK

Around the year 1380, the Dominican friar Henry Daniel composed his herbal, the *Aaron Danielis*, preserved in London, British Library, Additional MS 27329.[1] By that time the genre of pharmacological manuals had been developing for over one thousand years in Western Europe. Henry had a large corpus of herbals, antidotaries, glossaries, and learned medical commentaries to read for material and inspiration. Pharmacy during much of the early and central Middle Ages (ca. 500–1050 CE) was dominated by two works, the *Herbarius* of Apuleius Platonicus or "Pseudo-Apuleius" and the Latin translation of Dioscorides' *De materia medica* (the so-called *Dioscorides Longobardus*), but the later eleventh through fourteenth centuries saw the composition of dozens of new pharmacological texts. Henry Daniel's knowledge of herbs comes primarily from such high medieval "scholastic" or "Salernitan" herbals, those associated with the revival of learned medical theory in southern Italy around the port city of Salerno and the Abbey of Montecassino. Some of the defining features of the newer herbals are their translation or adaptation from classical Greek or medieval Arabic medical texts, the incorporation of previously unknown Asian herbs and spices into European pharmacy, and the application of Galen's system of pharmacological degrees to the substances discussed.[2]

Prominent among the newer pharmacological works cited in the *Aaron Danielis* are Constantine the African's *Liber graduum* (ca. 1080), the *Circa instans* attributed to Platearius (ca. 1150), the *Antidotarium Nicolai* (ca. 1140), the glossary known as *Alphita* (ca. 1200), and the books on plants from Bartholomaeus Anglicus's *De proprietatibus rerum* (ca. 1240). These pharmacological texts, and many others known to Henry Daniel, were written in Latin prose. Two key sources of the *Aaron Danielis* are, however, exceptional for having been written in Latin verse: *De viribus herbarum* of Macer Floridus and *Anglicanus Ortus* of Henry of Huntingdon.[3] In this essay I will examine Henry Daniel's techniques in translating and adapting these two works. He had to translate these works twice, in a sense: first from Latin into English and second from verse into prose. This process of double translation can sometimes reveal more of Henry Daniel's understanding of herbal medicine and his editorial choices than the often simpler translation of Latin prose into English. In his adaptations of the Latin herbal poems, we can see Henry Daniel making choices about what terms, phrases, and ideas he should translate carefully, which could be ignored, which censored, and which needed further explanation for his English audience.

## The Herbals of Macer Floridus and Henry of Huntingdon

The verse herbals of Macer Floridus and Henry of Huntingdon are significant representatives of a unique period in European education and literature. It was primarily in the period ca. 1075–1225 CE, the so-called long twelfth century, that a number of learned clerics in Europe wrote textbooks in Latin verse on topics as varied as grammar, theology, canon law, mathematics, and astronomy, as well as on medicine, pharmacy, and the virtues of stones.[4] These works are didactic in function and rarely deserve the name of poetry; their verses were mnemonic, helping students and scholars recall large amounts of technical information. While Latin didactic verse existed in the early Middle Ages (such as in Walahfrid Strabo's ninth-century CE work the *Hortulus*) and would continue to be written until the end of the medieval era, it was particularly during the long twelfth century that the genre flourished, especially in the form of medical poems.[5] Other didactic medical verses from this period are the *Regimen Sanitatis Salernitanum* (or *Flos medicinae*), composed around 1100 and enlarged by other medical poets throughout the rest of the later Middle Ages, and the medical verse treatises written by the French physician Gilles de Corbeil (ca. 1140–ca. 1220) in the later twelfth century.

"Macer" was the pseudonym adopted by a poet in the later eleventh century, generally agreed to be one Odo of Meung (Odo Magdunensis). As a native of Meung, Odo may have been a monk at the nearby abbey of Fleury in Orléans, a house with significant intellectual connections to Montecassino and thus access to the newest medical texts prepared at that abbey and in the nearby city of Salerno.[6] His *De viribus herbarum* ("On the Powers of Herbs," also known as *De virtutibus herbarum*, "On the virtues of herbs") is a Latin herbal in which each of seventy-seven herbs and spices is given its own poem describing the plant's medicinal properties (sixty-five European herbs and twelve Asian spices in the standard recension). The author is also known as Pseudo-Macer to distinguish him from the classical Roman poet Aemilius Macer (d. 16 BCE), whose name the medieval author borrowed. It seems that later scribes gave Pseudo-Macer the epithet *Floridus* ("flowery") and since then scholars have known both the author and his herbal as "Macer Floridus." Thanks to its memorable verses and accessible length, *De viribus herbarum* became one of the most popular herbals of the later Middle Ages. It survives in over 200 manuscript copies from the twelfth through sixteenth centuries, it was translated into every European vernacular language as well as Hebrew, and it was among the first European medical works to appear in print.[7] The herbal was so influential that any herbal of the later Middle Ages could be known as "a Macer."[8]

Due to its great popularity and open design, allowing for the easy addition or removal of lines and poems, Macer's herbal gained many imitators who wrote their own verse herbals or added new poems to *De viribus herbarum*. Some later medieval manuscripts of Macer Floridus include dozens or even hundreds more poems than the original seventy-seven, and these are frequently versifications of other prose herbals, such as the *Herbarius* of Pseudo-Apuleius or the *Circa instans*.[9] The most ambitious imitator of Macer Floridus was Henry, Archdeacon of Huntingdon (ca. 1088–ca. 1154), who wrote his own verse herbal *Anglicanus Ortus* ("The English Garden"), between the 1120s and 1140s. Henry of Huntingdon rewrote every one of the poems in *De viribus herbarum* and added nearly one hundred more new compositions to create an herbal of 160 poems organised into six books. He also wrote a Latin verse lapidary, or book on the virtues of stones, which he may have intended to accompany the herbal as part of a monumental medical verse treatise in eight books.[10]

Some of Henry of Huntingdon's poems are little more than reworded versions of Macer's poems, but he is often far more creative or "poetic" than Macer, as he provides personal reflections and favourite recipes and personifies some plants, addressing them as noisy characters in a comic drama. His herbal is representative of the classical revival of the Renaissance of the Twelfth Century, as Henry delights in fitting his medical knowledge into a pre-Christian, Mediterranean pagan setting: a potentially pagan *Natura* ("Mother Nature") grants healing powers to many plants, and the classical gods Apollo, Jupiter, and Clio make appearances to praise or criticise Henry, as narrator, and to imbue certain plants with healing virtue. *Anglicanus Ortus*, however, was not nearly as popular as *De viribus herbarum*, possibly because the poetic devices and characters actually interfered with the work's utility as an herbal. It survives in only one complete copy and partially in eight other manuscripts.[11] However, despite the relative rarity of *Anglicanus Ortus* in comparison to Macer's *De viribus herbarum*, Henry Daniel knew both of these verse herbals well and made their knowledge a key feature of the *Aaron Danielis*.

### Macer Floridus and Henry of Huntingdon in the *Aaron Danielis*: An Overview

The *Aaron Danielis* in Additional 27329 (ff. 4r–139v) contains approximately 800 separate headwords or entries. However, the majority of those entries are single lines, usually providing synonyms or cross-references to other entries; roughly 250 of the approximately 800 entries are longer and include cures and references to medical authorities. Henry Daniel incorporates information from the herbals of Macer Floridus, Henry of Huntingdon, or both in eighty-five of those approximately 250 longer entries, which demonstrates that their verse herbals were among his most important sources. Daniel uses fifty-two of the seventy-seven poems in *De viribus herbarum* (roughly two thirds of that work) and sixty-nine of the 160 poems from *Anglicanus Ortus* (at least 40 per cent).[12] A key difference between these numbers, however, which will be explained in greater detail below, is that Henry Daniel typically translates entire poems from *De viribus herbarum* but often merely refers to the presence of an herb in *Anglicanus Ortus* without translating the poem in question. This means that a much greater proportion of the *Aaron Danielis* is based directly on Macer's poems than on Henry of Huntingdon's.

Curiously, Henry Daniel did not use information from either verse herbal for a significant section at the start of *Aaron Danielis* (ff. 4r–26v, or over 16 per cent of the entire work), which includes all of letter A and about half of letter B. Most of the herbal poems that typically start with "A" in *De viribus herbarum* and *Anglicanus Ortus* are thus not translated or cited by Henry Daniel. Fifteen of Macer's twenty-five herbs that do not appear in the *Aaron Danielis* either begin with "A" in Macer's herbal or should have appeared under an "A" synonym in the *Aaron Danielis*.[13] Similarly, Henry Daniel does not use eleven herbs that start with "A" in *Anglicanus Ortus*.[14] The absence of these herbal poems from the *Aaron Danielis* is surprising given that they treat some of the most important examples of Eurasian *materia medica*, such as artemisia, wormwood, nettle, garlic, celery, mallow, dill, and sorrel (all of which begin with "A" in their most common Latin names). Granted, Henry Daniel still resorts to numerous other prose herbals for pharmaceutical remedies using these ingredients (primarily those of Platearius,

Constantinus Africanus, and Bartholomaeus Anglicus), but the absence of any information from *De viribus herbarum* or *Anglicanus Ortus* in these passages is striking and worth investigating.

There is no clear explanation for this lacuna in Additional 27329, especially given how eagerly Henry Daniel used the two verse herbals for the remainder of the *Aaron Danielis*. A potential answer is that Daniel simply did not have those herbals at first or did not want to use them when he began his work, but he obtained copies or changed his mind by the time he reached the middle of "B." Another possibility is that his source for the poems of Macer Floridus and Henry of Huntingdon was an alphabetical, composite herbal manuscript of their works that was acephalous and missing much of letters "A" and "B." Such a proposal is not too far-fetched given that the most complete English exemplar of *Anglicanus Ortus* is part of just such a composite, alphabetised herbal, found in London, British Library, Sloane MS 3468 (s.14), ff. 31r–105v. This alphabetical herbal is compiled from *De viribus herbarum*, the first four books of *Anglicanus Ortus*, and the prose *Herbarius* of Pseudo-Apuleius (here attributed to "Grosthede," i.e., Bishop Robert Grosseteste of Lincoln).[15]

Sloane 3468 also includes contemporary copies of the medical verses known as *Regimen Sanitatis Salernitanum* (ff. 6r–27r), Constantine the African's *De virtutibus simplicium medicinarum* (ff. 125r–136r), and a short treatise on weights and measures from the *Antidotarium Nicolai* (ff. 139v–142r), all of which Henry Daniel cites in his *Aaron Danielis*. While there is no indication that Henry Daniel knew of or used Sloane 3468 specifically, it seems likely he had on hand a similar composite manuscript. When considering what sort of manuscripts Henry Daniel used to compile the *Aaron Danielis*, we also have to consider his other, incomplete herbal in London, British Library Arundel MS 42 (it goes only up to the start of "G"). The Arundel 42 herbal includes most of the "A" entries from Macer Floridus and Henry of Huntingdon that were missing from Additional 27329.[16] While it is possible that Henry Daniel had an acephalous herbal compilation, it seems far more likely that he simply changed his mind between the composition of the two herbal recensions, deciding either to add or remove the information from those two verse herbals.

### Citation and Close Reading of Macer Floridus and Henry of Huntingdon

When translating the herbals of Macer Floridus and Henry of Huntingdon, Henry Daniel usually refers to the authors by name as "Macer" and "Henricus" or "Henricus Englisch." Daniel recognises that their works are closely related, with Henry of Huntingdon's poems nearly always treated as supplementary or additional to Macer's. Daniel usually gives credit to his sources whenever possible and forgets to name the verse herbalists in only a few cases. For example, in his entry "Borago" (borage, ff. 32vb–33rb), he translates all of Macer Floridus's "Barrocus" (lines 1641–63), but fails to name him (or perhaps his name was omitted by the scribe). However, Daniel does name Platearius before this passage and *Henricus Englisch* after it, so he is clearly trying to be open about his sources.

In 46 of the 85 entries drawing on the two verse herbals, Macer and Henry of Huntingdon are named together, with Macer always coming before Henry of Huntingdon. In nearly all of those cases (41 out of 46), Daniel translates the information in Macer's poem and then adds a sentence similar to "Henricus Englisch seith but þe same" (e.g., in "Brasica," f. 34vb). There is no entry in which Henry Daniel does the reverse, that is, in which he quotes at length from Henry of Huntingdon and simply notes that Macer says the same. At times Henry Daniel seems to grow tired of how often *Anglicanus Ortus* simply repeats the information found in *De viribus herbarum*. Daniel's lengthy entry "Betonica" (betony) is almost entirely a close translation of Macer's "Betonica" (lines 429–91). He ends this translation, "This seith Macer. Henricus Englisch seith but þe same, and therfore I preise not to put him" (f. 27rb).[17]

These patterns of translation and citation of the two verse herbals suggest that Henry Daniel had on hand separate and complete copies of *De viribus herbarum* and *Anglicanus Ortus*, or a composite herbal in which the authorship of individual poems was clearly indicated (as suggested above with reference to the herbal in Sloane MS 3468). What is clear is that for these 46 entries citing both Macer Floridus and Henry of Huntingdon, Daniel usually looked first in *De viribus herbarum* for his primary medical information and then compared the equivalent entry from *Anglicanus Ortus* to note any key differences. For example, in Daniel's entry "Borago" (borage), he concludes his translation of Macer's poem with the statement, "Henricus Englisch þe same, and he seith þe erbe ofte ete cureth toth ake" (f. 33rb). This suggests that Daniel closely read Henry of Huntingdon's poem "Boragum" and noted the one line ("Mansa diu dentis cladem reparat comedentis") that provided medical information not found in Macer's equivalent poem "Barrocum" (lines 1641–63).[18] Henry Daniel likewise translates Macer's poem on coriander, "Coriandrum" (lines 957–87), for his entry on the same (ff. 68va–69ra) and concludes that entry: "Henricus Englisch þe same, and this he addeth: if þu may not have peper, tak seed of coriandre, of carvi and cresse, and of percile, and þu schalt have saus ny off the same tast." Henry of Huntingdon adds culinary recipes like this several times to the material he found in Macer's herbal, and Henry Daniel recognised that this was new and useful information.[19]

A similar example of Henry Daniel's close comparison of the two verse herbals is seen in his entry on "Buglossa" (f. 37v), a case that gives some indication of the actual text in his source manuscripts and how it differed from the available modern editions. In this entry Daniel provides a close translation of Macer's "Buglossa" (lines 1127–38), after which he states: "If decocion of him be strowed and sperplied at mete among folk, it maketh hem alle blithe and glad; þe same seith Henricus Englisch, save þat Macer seith water, he seith lewk water; and Plinius seith þe same of Buglosse." Daniel here notes a difference between Macer's and Henry of Huntingdon's poems on the same herb, for he thought only the latter called for "lewk water."[20] The relevant line (1133) in Choulant's 1832 edition of Macer's *De viribus herbarum* does call for lukewarm (tepid) water, "Mixtus aquae tepidae si succus sumitur eius," but Henry Daniel does not seem to have had that version before him. Choulant notes that in some manuscripts line 1133 begins "Aquae frigidae succus …," and this reading may be what Henry Daniel had on hand when he claims that Macer called only for water where Henry of Huntingdon called for "lewk water" (*aque … tepide*). The final lines of Henry Daniel's "Buglossa" also show that some of his apparent sources came to him through other works. His reference to *Plinius* comes not from an actual work by Pliny the Elder or a later Pseudo-Pliny (such as the late-antique texts *Medicina Plinii* or *Physica Plinii*), but from Henry of Huntingdon's "Buglossa," which ends with a reference to Pliny.[21] This is only one of several instances in which Daniel cites authorities that reached him in this second-hand manner through his direct sources. In another example, Henry Daniel's "Iriginon" (f. 102v) is a translation of Macer's "Senecion" (lines 1664–89). Daniel refers twice in that entry to the opinions of "Plinius" about this herb, but both instances come directly from Macer. Or, similarly, Daniel's "Camomilla" (ff. 43rb–45ra) is based partly on Macer's "Chamomilla" (lines 549–91) with reference to Henry of Huntingdon's poem on the same (#1.13). Daniel seems to reach the end of his material from Macer when he says "thus Macer of anthemus" (an alternate name for chamomile) and then proceeds to outline a violet recipe attributed to "Plinius" (f. 44vb). But this attribution is misleading, because the following section under the name of Plinius is again translated directly from the end of Macer's poem (lines 580–91).

In only four instances does Henry Daniel use herbal information from Henry of Huntingdon and not from Macer, when the herb in question does have its own poem in *De viribus herbarum*: "Betoncion," "Bulbus Hastus," "Gliconius," and "Origanus."[22] The absence of Macer Floridus in these entries may again provide a clue to the specific manuscript of *De viribus herbarum* Henry Daniel used. Given that Daniel is otherwise conscientious and thorough in his translation of Macer's herbal, his manuscript may have been missing these specific poems. In just one instance does Henry Daniel use equivalent poems from the two verse herbals in separate entries of the *Aaron Danielis*: Henry of Huntingdon's poem on catnip, "Nepta" (#3.23), is based directly on Macer's "Nepeta" (lines 592–625). Both authors emphasise that *calamentum* is a synonym for *nepta/nepeta*, but Henry Daniel treats them as separate herbs, providing an entry "Calamenta" (ff. 41vb–42va) that uses Henry of Huntingdon's poem but not Macer's and an entry "Nepita" that does the reverse. But because Henry of Huntingdon's poem is essentially a verse "translation" of Macer's poem, Henry Daniel repeats all the same medical indications in his two entries.

In some cases, both Macer's and Henry of Huntingdon's herbals serve simply to add vocabulary, but not cures, to one of Henry Daniel's entries. Daniel's "Bisara" (rue, ff. 30ra–30va) is mostly a translation of Platearius' discussion of rue. But towards the end of "Bisara" Daniel says "Macer and Henricus Englisch seyn þat *piganon* grecus is 'rue' in Latyn." This comment demonstrates a close reading of both of their herbals, for this information is found only in one line (321) of both Macer's lengthy poem "Ruta" (lines 267–331) and Henry of Huntingdon's "Ruta" (*Anglicanus Ortus* #1.10, line 58). Daniel does not translate or cite any other lines in their poems on rue.

In only two entries ("Centauria" and "Eleborus") does Henry Daniel provide the names of both Macer and Henry of Huntingdon but no information from their works, instead saying, with reasonable accuracy, that the two authors say the same as the previously discussed authorities. For example, in "Centauria," Henry Daniel translates from *Alphita*, *Circa instans*, and Constantinus, after which he adds, "Bartholomeus reherceth þe same brefly; Macer and Henri Englisch eke." A tone of exhaustion is found in Daniel's entry "Eleborus" (hellebore), in which he states, "Macer and Henricus speken of elebre rigth prolix, but al þat thei seyn in prolixite Platearius seith it in brefte. Se in adarasto" (ff. 76vb–77ra). To be sure, Macer's and Henry of Huntingdon's respective poems on white and black hellebore are among their longest,[23] but Henry Daniel is not being entirely honest here. Platearius says rather different things about the hellebores and his entry is hardly brief, as can be seen in Henry Daniel's entry "Adarasta" (ff. 7ra–8ra), where he translates all of Platearius's lengthy passage on hellebore "word for word" (f. 8ra), and provides much more information not found in the standard edition of the *Circa instans*.[24]

In two other entries ("Butalmon" [better known as *plantago*, plantain] and "Elifagus" [better known as *salvia*, sage]) Henry Daniel gives the complete information from both Macer and Henry of Huntingdon, a clear indication that he generally considered just Macer sufficient when offered the choice of the same plant in both authors' works. Even in the case of "Butalmon," where most of Henry of Huntingdon's poem "Plantago" (#5.1.1) is translated, Henry Daniel makes the older Henry's work subservient to Macer's: "Henricus Englisch seith þe same poyntes save thus ..." (f. 38vb). Finally, there is only one entry, "Epithimus" (dodder of thyme, ff. 82rb–83vb), in which Henry Daniel names both Macer and Henry of Huntingdon, but the translated portion attributed to Macer does not come from the standard 77-poem recension of *De viribus herbarum*. I have not been able to identify a source for this passage in any of the later *spuria Macri*. Conversely, the portion of Henry Daniel's "Epithimus" that he attributes to "Henricus Englisch" actually comes from Henry of Huntingdon's poem "Thimus" (thyme, #6.2.26) and not his own poem "Epitimum" (#6.2.12). Clearly Henry Daniel was confused between the two plants and he notes at the start of his entry on "Epithimus" that he was not alone: "many auctoures as it semeth douten quat it is or quat it arn" (f. 82rb).

In the remaining thirty-nine entries under discussion, ten provide information from only Macer and twenty-nine from only Henry of Huntingdon. The significant difference can be explained by the fact that every poem in Macer's herbal has an equivalent poem in Henry of Huntingdon's, but *Anglicanus Ortus* contains nearly one hundred herbs and spices not found in *De viribus herbarum*. Henry Daniel seems to have had a complete version of *Anglicanus Ortus* in six books. This is a point worth remarking on because today the only surviving copy of the complete, six-book *Anglicanus Ortus* was written in Bohemia during the fifteenth century and remains to this day in Prague. Henry Daniel thus had a complete version of Henry of Huntingdon's herbal in fourteenth-century England, a copy that apparently no longer survives.[25]

### Henry Daniel's Translation of Latin Verse Herbals: Two Examples

I have provided a general overview of how Henry Daniel presents and cites the herbals of Macer Floridus and Henry of Huntingdon in his *Aaron Danielis*. In this section I will provide some detailed examples of

Table 1. Henry Daniel and Macer Floridus on Lettuce

| Henry Daniel, "Lactuca," *Aaron Danielis*, London, British Library Additional MS 27329, ff. 105vb–106ra | Macer Floridus, "Lactuca," *De viribus herbarum* #20, ll. 765–775 (ed. Choulant 1832), trans. Winston Black |
| --- | --- |
| **Lactuca**, lactusia, letuse: þer ben of 2 speces, tame & wylde; quan thou redest lactuca allone, undertond þe tame; thus Alphita. Macer: lactuca is cold and rigth moist. If it be ete, it abateth excessyf hetes; it doth þe same stamped wel & leyd to above. Also ete it is good for stomac & [106ra] disposeth to sleep and neschetz wombe; but in alle these it doth beter if it be ete soden, but to þe stomac is it beter if it be ete onwasched. The seed þerof letteth veyn dremyng, & drunk with wyn stauncheth wombe flux. If it be ete & drunk ofte time of þer noris it ʒeveth plente milk. Somme seyn if it be often used in etyn it apperreth sigth. Henricus þe same. ... [*After this come translations from "Platearius,""Avicenna," and "Diascorides" on the subject of lettuce.*] | Frigida Lactucae vis constat et humida valde, Unde potest nimios haec mansa levare calores, Et praestabit idem superaddas si bene tritam; Utilis est stomacho, somnum dat, mollit et alvum, Omnibus his melius prodest decocta comesta, Et stomacho potius non lota comesta medetur. Lactucae semen compescit somnia vana, Cum vino bibitum fluxum quoque reprimit alvi, Lac dat abundanter nutrici sumpta frequenter. Ut quidam dicunt oculis caligo creatur His, quibus assiduo fuerit cibus eius in usu. The power of Lettuce is very cold and moist, for which reason it is able, when eaten, to relieve excessive heat, and if you apply it, ground well, on top it will do the same thing. It is useful for the stomach, grants sleep, and softens the belly. It is better for all of these things to eat it cooked in water, but it heals the stomach better if it is eaten unwashed. Lettuce seed restrains empty dreams, and drunk with wine it also represses running of the belly [diarrhoea]. Eaten frequently it provides milk abundantly to a wetnurse. Some say that a cloudiness comes to the eyes of those who use [lettuce] frequently as food. |

how Daniel translated and adapted the individual Latin poems of these authors within his herbal. Tables 1 and 2 reproduce two of the entries in the *Aaron Danielis*, "Lavendula" and "Lactuca," on the left and the relevant passages from *De viribus herbarum* or *Anglicanus Ortus* on the right, with a modern English translation of the poem below. After each table I discuss how Henry Daniel incorporated the information from these Latin herbals into each respective entry. I have chosen these two examples because of their relative brevity and because they appear on the same folio towards the end of the herbal, at a point where Henry Daniel seems to have grown comfortable with his translation techniques. (Note that "L" does indeed come near the end of *Aaron Danielis*, because Henry Daniel provided noticeably fewer entries for herbs M-Z, found on folios 109b–139va.) When compared, they show some of the general trends in how Henry Daniel translated these two verse herbals differently.

Most of the longer entries in the *Aaron Danielis* begin with a list of synonyms and some, like *Lactuca*, include a distinction of types ("speces"). This information frequently comes from the *Alphita*, as noted here. Henry Daniel then typically launches into a translation of one of his major sources, here attributing his information to Macer. He closely translates Macer Floridus's poem on "Lactuca," repeating all of his specific preparations and indications for lettuce. However, in translating from the Latin verse, Henry Daniel makes a variety of small changes that modify the sense of the original. Where Macer says "The power [*vis*] of Lettuce is very cold and moist, For which reason it is able, when eaten, to relieve excessive heat," Henry Daniel renders this statement more simply as "lactuca is cold and rigth moist," but the meaning is not lost. However, Daniel's failure to translate Macer's *Unde* (line 766) removes a small but important key to the underlying natural philosophy: lettuce "abateth excessyf hetes" exactly because (*Unde*) it is very cold and moist. Daniel no doubt understood this connection but does not make it explicit for his English readers. Daniel also takes the liberty, probably unconscious, in his translation of Macer's line 773, according to which "eaten frequently it [lettuce] provides milk abundantly to a wetnurse." Daniel states that the plant can be "ete & drunk" by the nurse ("noris") for this effect. Daniel concludes his section on Macer with the accurate statement that "Henricus þe same," for Henry of Huntingdon's poem (#4.5) on lettuce is an abbreviated adaptation of Macer's poem and adds no new medical information.

For comparison with Henry Daniel's rendering of a poem by Macer Floridus, we can see in Table 2 how he translated and adapted a short poem by Henry of Huntingdon on the virtues of lavender. Macer does not treat this plant. Daniel is unsure about the identity of *lavendula* as he calls it a variety of (or similar to) sage (*salgia, elifagus*), liverwort (*epatica*), hyssop (*isope*), and rosemary.[26] While Henry of Huntingdon's poem does not describe lavender's appearance, his emphasis on the plant's redolent odour and use in protecting clothing and books clearly suggests the lavender we know to this day. In his translation of this poem, Henry Daniel is clear about his source ("Henricus writeth lavandula"), but he has done away with almost all of the more poetic or decorative elements of Henry of Huntingdon's writing. Where Henry of Huntingdon says, "Lavender, well-praised, is shining in her scented

Table 2. Henry Daniel and Henry of Huntingdon on Lavender

| Henry Daniel, "Lavendula," *Aaron Danielis*, London, British Library Additional MS 27329, f. 105va–vb | Henry of Huntingdon, "Lavandula," *Anglicanus Ortus* 1.8, (ed. and trans. Black 2012) |
| --- | --- |
| **Lavendula:** somme sey it is salvia or salgia minor, salvia silvestris, se in elifagus & in epatica; somme othere sey þe same, but thei sey it is mikil lyk isope, & is rigth hoot & migthy for þe palasy. But wite wel lavendula is þe femel of rosemaryn lavendre: se in ros marinus. Henricus writeth lavandula, & thus he seith: lauandle is a sote herbe-- ladies put it in her wyn, & clerkes in her bokes & clothes, boþe to kepe hem from wirmes & motthes & to do hem have good odor, for wyn {col b} or bokes or clothes þat it hatz lyn in, do it awey, & it kepe þe odor as thou it were stille þerin. In medicines it is on of þe gode herbis þat men fynde. | Fulget odorifero laudata lauandula lecto. Hanc peplis regina suis, hanc ponere gaudet Clericus in libris; hanc qui studio preciosas Conseruat uestes inponit uestibus ipsis. Hinc peplum, libri, uestes redolent ut ab ipsis Ipsam si demas, absens uideatur adesse. Hec dotes tantas tanto contraxit odore Vt si mater ei uires Natura dedisset In medicamentis nichil equum tradere quisquam Posse uidetur. Vix ergo superba medetur.

Lavender, well-praised, is shining in her scented bed. A queen rejoices to place this inside her royal robes, a cleric inside his books; one who would keep with care his precious garments enfolds this in his clothes. Robes and books and clothing are so redolent of it, that if you take away the herb, when absent it still seems present there. It has drawn together such great gifts with so great an odour that if Mother Nature had endowed it with some powers in medicine, it seems no one could supply its equal. Therefore haughty, she can scarcely heal. |

bed," Henry Daniel simply states "lauandule is a sote herbe." According to Henry of Huntingdon, the queen (perhaps Matilda of Scotland, wife of Henry I of England, who died in 1118, and whom Henry of Huntingdon knew well and admired) put lavender in her robes. Henry Daniel reduces the queen in rank to "ladies" and he renders the Latin *peplis* ("robes") as "wine." Daniel likewise leaves out the word *peplum* in his translation of line 5 of this poem. This apparently incorrect translation suggests that Daniel was reading a copy of *Anglicanus Ortus* more like the manuscript Sloane 3468, of English provenance, than the complete copy Prague, Knihovna metropolitní kapituly, ms M. VI 1359, copied in Bohemia. For in Sloane 3468, the poem on lavender contains *prelis* for *peplis* in line 2 and *preli* for *peplum* in line 5.[27] A *prelum* is a wine-press, which can stand through synecdoche for wine itself or a winecup. It is unlikely that Daniel's translation to "wine" stems from confusion about the word *peplis*, for not long after this point in the *Aaron Danielis* he distinguishes the neuter noun *peplum* from the masculine *peplus*: "Peplus is a spece of thistil in quich crop growe smale heres. þat at litil steryng it flie awey in þe eyr. It is þe blac thistil. And peplum is velamen mulierum womman veyl" (f. 119va). I have not found a source for this definition of *peplus*, which could be an alternate spelling of *pepilus*, tentatively identified by Tony Hunt as common windgrass rather than as a species of thistle.[28]

Yet Daniel also elaborates on some of Henry of Huntingdon's poem, for he explains exactly why clerics put lavender in their books and vestments: "boþe to kepe hem from wirmes and motthes and to do hem have good odor." Henry of Huntingdon no doubt understood that point, but merely states in his poem that books and clothing pleasantly retain the odour of lavender. Daniel both dramatically shortens and misunderstands Henry of Huntingdon's last four lines of this poem, in which the archdeacon stressed that lavender actually is not useful in medicine: "It has drawn together such great gifts with so great an odour/that if Mother Nature had endowed it with some powers/in medicine, it seems no one could supply/its equal. Therefore haughty, she can scarcely heal."[29] If Henry Daniel had before him lines 7–10 of this poem as they appear in the surviving manuscripts, he clearly did not understand the Latin, for he renders this passage simply as "In medicines it is on of þe gode herbis þat men fynde" (f. 105v), a statement that contradicts Henry of Huntingdon's argument. Of course, it is possible that Daniel simply disagreed with Henry of Huntingdon, for he understood lavender to be a type of either sage or rosemary, both of which were used extensively in later medieval herbal medicine.[30] Whether or not Henry Daniel understood the main point of these final lines, they also demonstrate some of his usual tendencies in translating Henry of Huntingdon's poems: Daniel has not translated either the attribution of the plant's virtues to *mater Natura* or the personification of the plant itself as *superba* ("haughty"). These poetic turns are typical of *Anglicanus Ortus*, but Henry Daniel has no interest in replicating them in his more pragmatic herbal.

### Translating Macer Floridus and Henry of Huntingdon: General Trends

The specific examples of lettuce and lavender give some indication of how Henry Daniel approached the translation and adaptation of the Latin verse herbals of Macer Floridus and Henry of Huntingdon. In this final section I will outline some of the more general trends that can be observed in his translations from Latin verse to Middle English prose. Already it should be clear that "translation" for Henry Daniel is often not a word-for-word process, even when he frequently claims to be doing that in both the *Aaron Danielis* and his *Liber Uricrisiarum*.[31] From the start of his herbal, Henry Daniel's main concern is to create a straightforward catalogue of the medicinal effects and therapeutic uses of common and exotic plants. For this reason, he is typically more faithful in his translations of Macer than of Henry of Huntingdon because Macer's poems contain almost entirely pharmacological information without any of Henry of Huntingdon's poetic indulgences. As noted above, when Daniel cites Macer he usually translates the entire poem, often word for word or at least line by line. If any elements are missing from Macer's account, it is most likely because Daniel missed them or the relevant lines were lacking from his manuscript of *De viribus herbarum*.

The most notable changes that Henry Daniel makes to Macer's entries occur when he interjects a definition or brief comment on an important term. For example, Daniel's entry "Betonica" (betony, ff. 26va–27rb) is almost entirely a close translation of Macer's poem "Betonica" (lines 429–91). However, when Macer calls for *cyathis tribus* of wine in a recipe, Daniel translates this and then adds, "Ciatus and aureus is 12 peny wight" (f. 27ra), providing his English readers with a better understanding of these technical terms of Greek origin. Likewise, in his entry "Ligustra" (ff. 107vb–108rb) he translates Macer's poem "Ligusticum" (lines 882–906), but interrupts his translation with a reference to his other composition, the uroscopic manual *Liber Uricrisiarum*, for more information on a technical term in Macer's poem.[32] Where Macer says that lovage seed is good in all antidotes helping digestion,[33] Henry Daniel adds a cross-reference to his other work where he explains the process of digestion: "If it be drunk his seed in alle medicines þat helpe þe digestion. Off 3 digestions, se in oure speculatyf of Uricrisis" (f. 108ra). This addition obviously will not help the casual reader of the herbal understand the body's three digestions, but if their library holds the *Liber Uricrisiarum* they will know where to look.[34] Daniel also makes additions to his translation of Macer that provide a religious connection, not unsurprising given his vocation as a Dominican friar. Much of Daniel's entry "Pastinaca" (parsnip, ff. 118vb–119rb) is a translation of Macer's "Pastinaca" (lines 1264–84). Macer explains at the end of his poem that *pastinaca* is so named because it is the best root for food (*pastum*).[35] Daniel clearly was taken with this passage because he moved it to the start of his own entry (he rarely reorganises the poems he translates in this fashion) and in between two lines translated from Macer he adds the claim that John the Baptist lived on parsnips: "And therfore seith Macer beter fode to man ʒeveth no rote than this. Be this rote s. Jon Baptist lived most by in wildirnes Macer for it ȝeveth fode it is cald pastenep" (ff. 118vb–119ra).

Even though Macer Floridus usually provided exactly the sort of medical information that Henry Daniel wanted in his own herbal, there were times when Henry Daniel felt he could significantly abbreviate his translation of *De viribus herbarum*. This often occurred in the opening lines of poems, where Macer is sometimes more discursive. Henry Daniel's entry "Lapaphus" (dock, ff. 106vb–107ra) is a translation of Macer's "Paratella" (lines 1993–2014). He translates Macer's first four lines (1993–6) on the varieties and virtues of dock with just nine words: "þer ben 3 speces, and alle hot and dry." In a similar case, Daniel dramatically shortens the opening five lines of Macer's poem "Porrum" (leek, lines 507–48) in his entry "Prassus" (ff. 122va–123ra) and strips them of some complexity. Macer explains that Hippocrates prescribed a drink of leek juice to patients who spat up blood, called *haemoptoicos* in Greek.[36] Daniel removes any mention of the technical term for this condition as well as Macer's epithet for Hippocrates as "the greatest founder of medicine," and renders this passage more simply as "And ipocras ȝaf this herbe to a thousand folk þat spitteden blood and it halp hem." However, it is curious that Daniel specifies "a thousand folk" when Macer does not give a number.

A more dramatic abbreviation of Macer's text occurs in Daniel's "Pionia" (peony, ff. 120rb–120vb), which is primarily an adaptation of Macer's "Paeonia" (lines 1605–40). Macer gives a lengthy description in eleven lines (1617–27) of an experiment supposedly performed by Galen, in which he hung a peony root around the neck of an eight-year-old boy with epilepsy. As long as the boy wore the root he suffered no attacks, but as soon as Galen removed it, the boy immediately collapsed in an epileptic fit. Henry Daniel abbreviates this passage to the briefer statement, "Rote of pian [i.e., peony] hangid about þe nek of childre þat have þe epilence it is helpe to hem. And Galien telleth how he tooke þe rote fro þe nek of a chyld þat had þe epilence and he fel and he dede it ageyn and þe child ros in good poynt." Daniel retains the essentials of Macer's passage here, but it is no longer a translation. Rather, he has rephrased sections of Macer's poem in his own idiom, meaning not just a different language but a different tone and level of detail.

Whereas the preceding examples show Henry Daniel cutting what he saw as extraneous verbiage from his translation, while retaining the essential meaning of the passage in Macer, there are some cases where he actively censors subjects in Macer's herbal. This occurs especially in the case of birth control remedies and abortifacients, subjects that did not bother Macer or Henry of Huntingdon. Macer's poem on mint,

"Mentha" (lines 1569–84), instructs a woman to insert mint juice in her vagina before intercourse so that she may prevent conception.[37] In his entry "Menta" (ff. 111ra–112ra) Daniel translates all of Macer's poem closely but skips over the final two lines on this subject. There is no indication that any manuscripts are missing this passage, so it seems that Daniel consciously made this omission. Similarly, Macer's poem "Ostrutium" (lines 907–27) provides a recipe for an abortifacient and an emmenagogue for a delayed period,[38] which Daniel cuts from his translation in "Ostricion" (f. 117va). There are numerous other instances where Daniel does translate abortifacients from Macer's herbal, but those are clearer about bringing out a dead foetus rather than aborting a viable foetus, which is suggested here in these two passages from Macer.

In another case Henry Daniel has rewritten Macer's herbal apparently to transform an aphrodisiac into an anaphrodisiac. Macer's poem "Prassus," already discussed above, features a recipe in which a leek, eaten raw, alleviates drunkenness, stimulates sexual desire (*venerem*), and softens a hard belly.[39] Daniel translates this passage in an apparently straightforward manner: "If it be ete raw abateth dronkinhede and abateth þe lecchere and nescheth hard wombe." It is difficult to tell whether Daniel intended to change the meaning of Macer's poem. The incorrect translation of Macer's *stimulat* may be due simply to the accidental repetition of the verb *abateth* and, what is more, there are several other instances in the *Aaron Danielis* where Henry Daniel was not ashamed to translate an aphrodisiac recipe from his Latin source.[40]

In his quest to compile a comprehensive and functional herbal, Henry Daniel actively removed the more poetic passages from his translations of Macer Floridus and Henry of Huntingdon. He refused to translate most lines from their works with classical images, historical references, metaphors, or descriptions of beauty. Such lines are far more common in Henry of Huntingdon's *Anglicanus Ortus* but Macer occasionally indulged in such poetic licence too. He begins his poem on violets ("Violae," lines 1342–94) with the statement that "Neither the splendor of roses nor lilies can overcome the fragrant violets in appearance, strength, or odor" (lines 1342–3: "Nec roseus superare decor, nec lilia possunt / Fragrantes Violas specie, nec vi, nec odore"). Henry Daniel does not include this statement in his translation, found in the lengthy entry "Bisaco" (ff. 28r–30r), an alternate name for the more usual *viola*. Henry of Huntingdon, with his usual poetic flair, says that if a person eats the seed of "Cicuta" (hemlock, #5.1.11), "you will be conquered, loving Venus and bitter Love."[41] Henry Daniel translates most of Henry of Huntingdon's poem in his entry "Benedicta" but renders this passage simply as "it stauncheth lecchere" (f. 26va).

Henry Daniel's pruning of the poems of Henry of Huntingdon is more dramatic, as he frequently ignores or simplifies numerous lines in *Anglicanus Ortus* that do not fit his vision for the *Aaron Danielis*. Daniel removes from his translations of *Anglicanus Ortus* references to classical sources: Pliny disappears from Daniel's "Bulbus Hastus" (ff. 37r–37v) when he is named explicitly in his source, Henry of Huntingdon's "Sempervivum" (#3.25, line 3), and Daniel removes Anaxialus from his translation of Henry of Huntingdon's "Cicuta" (#5.1.11) in his entry "Benedicta" (ff. 26r–26v). Daniel similarly removes most references to classical stories and divinities, which are relatively common in *Anglicanus Ortus*. He translates most of Henry of Huntingdon's "Apium" (#1.20) in his entry "Betoncion" (f. 27v) but ignores all of the first eleven lines of the poem, in which we learn that ancient warriors wore this plant on their helmets after a victory, a tradition supposedly begun by Hercules. Daniel ignores Henry of Huntingdon's statement that the muse Calliope sang about the virtues of herbs, when translating his "Lappa" (#5.1.12) in his entry "Caballus marinus" (f. 41r), and he likewise cuts from his "Calamenta" (ff. 42r–42v) Henry of Huntingdon's reference to wine as the "drink of Bacchus," not even translating it simply as wine.[42]

Henry Daniel is especially ruthless in cutting most of Henry of Huntingdon's elaborate double poem "Iacinctus et Narcissus" (#4.1–2), in which he describes in verse the legends of how the flowers hyacinth and narcissus are named after the ancient youths Iacinctus and Narcissus. Henry Daniel translates in "Iacinctus" (ff. 101r–101v) only eight of the poem's thirty-six lines, namely those that directly concern the medicinal virtues of hyacinth. Yet Daniel's unfamiliarity with classical myth comes through in this passage, for he wrongly understands "Elicon" as a synonym for "iacinctus," when it is actually the place in Greece where Narcissus was born, Mount Helicon.

As we saw above in the case of "Lavandula," Henry Daniel did not translate Henry of Huntingdon's reference to *Natura*, who is a prominent figure in *Anglicanus Ortus*. Daniel seems to have systematically ignored any reference to this autonomous, potentially pagan figure. In his "Crocus" (f. 70vb) he also ignores the description of *Natura parens* ("Mother Nature") endowing the crocus with powers to fight disease (from Henry of Huntingdon, "Crocus," #1.3, line 12). Henry Daniel's concerns about *Natura* are made especially clear in his translation of Henry of Huntingdon's "Plantago" (#5.1.1) in his "Butalmon" (ff. 38vb–39v), in which he renders the Latin "Omnipotens ... natura" (#5.1.1, line 1) as "almigthi God" (f. 38vb). Of course, according to Christian theology and philosophy this translation is not wholly incorrect, as "nature" could rightly be seen as the action of God in time, but the fact that Henry Daniel consistently ignores or changes *Natura* suggests a discomfort on his part with this personification. In a similar act of quiet censorship in his entry on "Gliconius" (ff. 97r–97v), Henry Daniel changes Henry of Huntingdon's statement in his poem "Pulegium" (#2.16) that the "marvelous virtue of the Thunderer" (i.e., Jupiter) granted virtuous plants to every region of the world.[43] Daniel instead says that "men seye þat pulole is deynte in þe lond of Ynde as peper is among us" (f. 97va). This change is noteworthy because Daniel otherwise translates relatively carefully every other line of this poem and it suggests that he was again uncomfortable with attributing divine actions to a non-Christian deity.

A study of Henry Daniel's incorporation of the verse herbals of Macer Floridus and Henry of Huntingdon into his *Aaron Danielis* does not concern just translation from Latin into Middle English. Daniel's processes of "translation" involved the careful reading of their poems to discern the elements most important for his own herbal, the critical comparison and juxtaposition of related poems in those two works, and the muting or censorship of poetic and classical themes that were dangerous or unworthy of a work of Dominican scholarship. Irma Taavitsainen remarked, concerning Daniel's composition of his *Liber Uricrisiarum*, "Henry Daniel's text builds upon passages quoted from various authorities, comparing them but keeping the discourse under control by frequent metatext and by presenting the commentator's own opinions."[44] This statement is equally true of the *Aaron Danielis*: Daniel crafted a new kind of pharmaceutical treatise for an English audience through the judicious pruning, pragmatic translation, and careful ordering of a large selection of Latin herbal texts. Daniel's use of every one of the Latin sources of the *Aaron Danielis* deserves further study, of course. What separates the herbals of Macer Floridus and Henry of Huntingdon from the rest of these sources is that Henry Daniel had to undertake several more stages of translation, selection, and adaptation to fit their didactic verse into his own pharmaceutical prose.

NOTES

1   This essay will address primarily the herbal in Additional 27329, which has no contemporary title but which a later hand calls *Aaron Danielis*. That manuscript also contains on ff. 140r–236r Henry Daniel's alphabetical list of other botanical and medical (that is, non-herbal) terms from *Abies* to *Zoib*. Daniel also began an alternate version of his herbal in London, British Library, Arundel MS 42, which contains information from both

the herbal and non-herbal catalogues in Additional 27329. It is not clear which version of the herbal came first. My thanks to Tess Tavormina, Ruth Harvey, Sarah Star, and Emily Reiner for their advice and suggestions on improving this chapter.

2 On these subjects, see the essays in *La Scuola Medica Salernitana. Gli autori e i testi*, ed. Danielle Jacquart and Agostino Paravicini Bagliani (Florence: SISMEL/Edizioni 2007) and *La* Collectio Salernitana *di Salvatore De Renzi*, ed. Danielle Jacquart and Agostino Paravicini Bagliani (Florence: SISMEL/Edizioni 2008), in particular Monica H. Green, "Rethinking the Manuscript Basis of Salvatore De Renzi's *Collectio Salernitana*: The Corpus of Medical Writings in the 'Long' Twelfth Century," in *La* Collectio Salernitana *di Salvatore De Renzi*, 15–60.

3 The standard editions are *Macer Floridus de Viribus Herbarum una cum Walafridi Strabonis, Othonis Cremonensis et Ioannis Folcz Carminibus similis argumenti ...*, ed. L. Choulant (Leipzig: Leopold Voss, 1832), 1–123, and Henry of Huntingdon, *Anglicanus Ortus: A Verse Herbal of the Twelfth Century*, ed. and trans. Winston Black. Studies and Texts 180. British Writers of the Middle Ages and Early Modern Period 3 (Toronto: Pontifical Institute of Mediaeval Studies; Oxford: Bodleian Library, 2012).

4 On the last subject, see the verse lapidary of Marbode of Rennes: Marbodus Redonensis, *Liber Lapidum. Lapidario*, ed. and trans. Maria Esthera Herrera (Paris: Les Belles Lettres, 2005). Marbode's lapidary was frequently copied together with Macer's herbal and the two texts circulated together as a verse compendium of natural and medical knowledge. See *Marbode of Rennes' (1035–1123) De lapidibus*, John M. Riddle and trans. C.W. King (Wiesbaden: Franz Steiner, 1977). The two works were so closely linked that the early modern editor Ianus Cornarius published Marbode's lapidary without attribution as the fifth book of a spurious five-book herbal attributed to Macer: *Macri, De materia medica, libri V* (Frankfurt: F.C. Egenhalf, 1540).

5 On the subject of medieval didactic poetry, primarily in Latin, see Lynn Thorndike, 'Unde Versus,' *Traditio* 11 (1955), 163–93; Vivien Law, "Why write a verse grammar?" *Journal of Medieval Latin* 9 (1999), 46–76; Jan Ziolkowski, "From Didactic Poetry to Bestselling Textbooks in the Long Twelfth Century," in *Calliope's Classroom: Studies in Didactic Poetry from Antiquity to the Renaissance*, ed. Annette Harder, Alasdair A. MacDonald, and Gerrit J. Reinink (Leuven: Peeters, 2007), 221–44; Winston Black, "Teaching the Mnemonic Bishop in the Medieval Canon Law Classroom," in *Envisioning the Bishop: Images and the Episcopacy in the Middle Ages*, ed. Evan Gatti and Sigrid Danielson (Turnhout: Brepols, 2014), 377–404.

6 Monica H. Green explores the possible contexts for the composition and patronage of *De viribus herbarum* in "Medicine in France and England in the Long Twelfth Century: Inheritors and Creators of European Medicine," in *France et Angleterre: manuscrits médiévaux entre 700 et 1200*, ed. Charlotte Denoël and Francesco Siri, *Bibliologia* 57 (Turnhout: Brepols, 2020), 365–90. For a broader study of Macer's intellectual milieu, see also Monica H. Green, "Medical Books," in *The European Book in the Twelfth Century*, ed. Erik Kwakkel and Rodney Thomson (Cambridge: Cambridge University Press, 2018), 277–92.

7 This number comes from my personal research into the manuscript tradition of *De viribus herbarum*.

8 A famous example is the Middle English herbal of John Lelamour found in British Library, Sloane MS 5, in which Lelamour claims to have translated the herbal of "Macer the philizofur." The herbal is not in fact based on Macer's *De viribus herbarum*. See David Moreno Olalla, *Lelamour Herbal (MS Sloane 5, ff. 13r–57r). An Annotated Critical Edition* (Bern: Peter Lang, 2018).

9 These additional poems were christened *Spuria Macri* by Ludwig Choulant in his edition of *De viribus herbarum* and some of the *spuria* are discussed at length by Ulrike Jansen in *"Spuria Macri": Ein Anhang zu "Macer Floridus, De viribus herbarum." Einleitung, Übersetzung, Kommentar* (Berlin: De Gruyter, 2013). However, see my review of this book in *Speculum* 90:1 (2015), 260–3.

10 There is no surviving manuscript of this work in eight books, but see my discussion of the manuscripts in Winston Black, "Henry of Huntingdon's Lapidary Rediscovered and his *Anglicanus Ortus* Reassembled," *Mediaeval Studies* 68 (2006), 43–87.

11 The only complete manuscript of the six-book herbal is Prague, Knihovna metropolitní kapituly, ms M. VI 1359, ff. 1r–47v, written in 1443 in or near Prague. That manuscript and four other witnesses are described in detail in Henry of Huntingdon, *Anglicanus Ortus*, 59–63. Since publishing my edition of *Anglicanus Ortus*, I have discovered four other witnesses to Henry of Huntingdon's poems, in all of which some of Henry's poems are compiled with Macer Floridus's *De viribus herbarum*: London, British Library, Sloane MS 2481 (1470–1480, German); London, British Library, Royal MS 12 B xii (s.13, England); London, British Library, Royal MS 12 E xxiii (s. 13[ex], southern England); Oxford, Bodleian Library, Digby MS 29 (s.14, England).

12 By all indications, Henry Daniel was translating directly from the standard Latin version of *De viribus herbarum*. But it would be useful to compare how Henry Daniel translated Macer Floridus to the translation

methods in the better-known Middle English version of Macer's herbal edited by Gösta Frisk (*A Middle English Translation of Macer Floridus de Viribus Herbarum*, Uppsala: Almqvist & Wiksells, 1949). Martti Mäkinen has begun this process in a recent essay, comparing that Middle English Macer with several Middle English recipe collections: "Herbal recipes and recipes in herbals – intertextuality in early English medical writing," in *Medical and Scientific Writing in Late Medieval English*, ed. Irma Taavitsainen and Päivi Pahta (Cambridge: Cambridge University Press, 2004), 144–73.

13   Those fifteen poems in *De viribus herbarum* are "Artemisia," "Abrotanum," "Absinthium," "Urtica" (called "Acalifa" by Daniel), "Allium," "Apium," "Althaea," "Anethum," "Acidula," "Portulaca" (called "Andrago" by Daniel), "Atriplex," "Aristolochia," "Iris" (called "Acorus" by Daniel), "Asarum," and "Aloe" (#1–5, #8–10, #18–19, #28, #41, #43, #46, #77 according to the numbering of Choulant's edition).

14   "Arthemisia" (#1.1), "Ambrosia" (#1.6), "Azimum" (#2.4), "Abrotanus" (#2.23), "Anetum" (#3.3), "Asarum" (#3.6), "Absinthium" (#3.11), "Altea" (#3.16), "Aristologia" (#4.23), "Aloe" (#6.1.12), "Anacardus" (#6.2.27) according to the numbering of Black's 2012 edition.

15   For more on this manuscript see Henry of Huntingdon, *Anglicanus Ortus*, 59.

16   In Arundel 42 Henry Daniel uses both Macer and Henry of Huntingdon's poems for his entries *Absynthyus*, *Abrotanus*, *Acalifa* (called *Urtica* in both verse herbals), *Ambrosia*, and *Arthemisia*; he uses just Henry of Huntingdon's poems for *Agaricus* and *Anetus*; but he still does not use either herbal for *Aloe*, *Asarus*, and *Aristologia*.

17   All quotations from the *Aaron Danielis* come from a transcription prepared by Dr. E. Ruth Harvey of the University of Toronto with revisions by Dr. M. Teresa Tavormina of Michigan State University. I am grateful to both of them for sharing their work with me. A critical edition is currently in preparation.

18   Henry of Huntingdon, "Boragum," *Anglicanus Ortus* #4.22, line 6 (ed. Black), 252.

19   On Henry of Huntingdon's culinary recipes see Winston Black, "Scenes from an Anglo-Norman Kitchen, Part 1: Mutton, Parsley, and Pagan Gods," *The Recipe Project* Oct. 13, 2016, https://recipes.hypotheses. org/8550, and Winston Black, "Scenes from an Anglo-Norman Kitchen, Part 2: Vegetable Cures and a Drunken Cook," *The Recipe Project* Nov. 3, 2016, https://recipes.hypotheses.org/8588.

20   Henry of Huntingdon, "Buglossa," *Anglicanus Ortus* #1.14, line 5 (ed. Black), 108: "Mixtus aque succus tepide si sumitur herbe …"

21 Henry of Huntingdon, "Buglossa," *Anglicanus Ortus* #1.14, lines 13–14 (ed. Black), 108:
  Plinius affirmat hoc, quod decoccio reddat
  Letos conuiuas hac si conuiuia spargas.

22 Henry Daniel, "Betoncion" (ff. 27vb–28rb), uses Henry of Huntingdon, "Apium" (#1.20), instead of Macer, "Apium" (lines 332–65); Henry Daniel, "Bulbus Hastus" (ff. 37rb–37va), uses Henry of Huntingdon, "Semperviva" (#3.25), instead of Macer, "Acidula" (lines 711–47); Henry Daniel, "Gliconius" (ff. 97ra–98ra), uses Henry of Huntingdon, "Pulegium" (#2.16), instead of Macer, "Pulegium" (lines 626–77); Henry Daniel, "Origanus" (ff. 116ra–117ra), uses Henry of Huntingdon, "Origanum" (#1.7), instead of Macer, "Origanum" (lines 1285–1324).

23 Macer Floridus, "Elleborus albus" and "Elleborus niger," *De viribus herbarum* #56–7, ll. 1774–1832, 1833–1858 (ed. Choulant 1832), 101–5. Henry of Huntingdon "Elleborum album" and "Elleborum nigrum," *Anglicanus Ortus* #2.2–2.3 (ed. Black 2012), 134–7.

24 "De elleboro," in *Das Arzneidrogenbuch Circa instans in einer Fassung des XIII. Jahrhunderts aus der Universitätsbibliothek Erlangen*, ed. Hans Wölfel (Berlin, 1939), 51. There are many small differences between Platearius' account of hellebore and the two poems on the hellebores found in Macer's herbal (and in Henry of Huntingdon's, which is based directly on Macer's poems). Platearius cites the authority of Dioscorides while Macer refers to Pliny and Themison. Platearius also names many more specific illnesses than Macer does, providing remedies for "melancoliam … et quartanam … artheticam, podagram et cyragram," etc.

25 It is worth pondering whether this was the very manuscript which served as the exemplar for the complete six-book *Anglicanus Ortus* found in Prague, Knihovna metropolitní kapituly, ms M. VI 1359. In my edition of that work, I suggest that "*P* … may owe its existence to a Bohemian scholar who accompanied Anne of Bohemia to England at the time of her marriage to Richard II in 1382, and carried the text from England back to his homeland after Richard's death. This is evidently the case with manuscripts of John Wycliffe's works." *Anglicanus Ortus*, 57. That must remain speculation without further manuscript discoveries, but Kristen L. Geaman lends credence to this point in her essay, "Anne of Bohemia and Her Struggle to Conceive," *Social History of Medicine* 29:2 (2016): 224–44, at 230.

26 Henry Daniel's cross-references send the reader on a wild goose chase in an attempt to understand this herb: He refers the reader to his entries on "Elifagus" and "Epatica." The confusion is increased when Daniel

states confidently ("wite wel") that *lavendula* is the female of the rosemary plant. Yet if we turn to his brief entry on "Rosmarinus" (f. 126v), there is no mention of lavender and he then points the reader to his much longer entry "Anthos" (ff. 16r–18r). At the very end of this entry (f. 18r), Daniel concludes "The female to him is lavendula: lyk in stok and schortere, and more qwyt. Floures depe blo and not so vertuous; but as qwyt fenel to þe rede fenell, or qwyt rose to þe red rose, nevertheles it is wol migthy to manye thingges. Se more in Rosmarinus."

    This confusion is all the more surprising as Henry Daniel was somewhat of an expert on rosemary. This lengthy passage on "Anthos" about the virtues of rosemary circulated separately from the *Aaron Danielis*, surviving in at least ten manuscripts. See also Martti Mäkinen, "Henry Daniel's Rosemary in MS X.90 of the Royal Library, Stockholm," *Neuphilologische Mitteilungen* 103:3 (2002), 305–27, and George R. Keiser, "Rosemary: Not Just for Remembrance," in *Health and Healing from the Medieval Garden*, ed. Peter Dendle and Alain Touwaide (Woodbridge: The Boydell Press, 2008), 180–204.

27  Henry of Huntingdon, *Anglicanus Ortus, apparatus* to I.8, p. 92.

28  Tony Hunt, *Plant Names of Medieval England* (Cambridge: D.S. Brewer, 1989), *s.v.* "Pepilus."

29  Henry of Huntingdon, "Lavandula," *Anglicanus Ortus* 1.8, lines 7–10 (ed. and trans. Black 2012), 95.

30  Daniel kept an open mind when reading and citing older medical works. He often disagreed with his sources in his *Liber Uricrisiarum*, as described by E. Ruth Harvey and M. Teresa Tavormina, "Introduction," in *Henry Daniel, Liber Uricrisiarum: A Reading Edition* (University of Toronto Press, 2020); and Sarah Star, "The Textual Worlds of Henry Daniel," *Studies in the Age of Chaucer* 40 (2018): 191–216, at 199–203.

31  Päivi Pahta and Irma Taavitsainen, "Vernacularisation of scientific and medical writing in its sociohistorical context," in *Medical and Scientific Writing in Late Medieval English*, ed. Irma Taavitsainen and Päivi Pahta (Cambridge University Press, 2004), 1–18, at 14. For examples of Daniel's assertions that he is translating a given passage almost *verbatim* ("nerhonde word for word"), see *Liber Uricrisiarum* 2.2.257, 2.2.306, 2.13.394, and elsewhere throughout the text.

32  Henry Daniel has confused Macer's *ligusticum* (lovage), an alternate spelling of *levisticum*, with *ligustrum*, which he identifies as "wyld lilie … liga, bynde" (f. 107vb).

33  Macer Floridus, *De viribus herbarum*, lines 898–9 (ed. Choulant):
      Digestibilibus semen bene iungitur eius
      Omnibus antidotis, quod inest sibi peptica virtus.

34  Henry Daniel describes the three digestions in his *Liber Uricrisiarum* I.3.

35  Macer Floridus, *De viribus herbarum*, lines 1283–4 (ed. Choulant):
    Quod pastum tribuat est Pastinaca vocata,
    Namque cibum nullae radices dant meliorem.
36  Macer Floridus, *De viribus herbarum*, lines 507–11 (ed. Choulant):
    In multis causis usus medicamine Porri
    Dicitur Ippocras, medicinae maximus auctor,
    Istius succum solum dedit ille Bibendum
    Aegrotis, qui reiiciunt sputantve cruorem,
    Quos haemoptoicos soliti sunt dicere Graeci ...
37  Macer Floridus, *De viribus herbarum*, lines 1581–2 (ed. Choulant):
    Matrici succus si subditur illius, ante
    Quam fiat coitus, mulier non concipit inde.
38  Macer Floridus, *De viribus herbarum*, lines 915–16 (ed. Choulant):
    Subdita matrici depellere fertur abortum,
    Et sic tarda nimis educere menstrua tradunt ...
39  Macer Floridus, *De viribus herbarum*, lines 547–8 (ed. Choulant):
    Si crudum fuerit sumptum levat ebrietatem,
    Sic venerem stimulat, sic duram mollit et alvum.
    Another explanation for the different description in *Aaron Danielis* is
    that Henry Daniel's manuscript of Macer read "Nec" instead of "Sic" in
    line 548, a common scribal error.
40  "Antophilus" (cloves) "maketh migthy to lecchere" (f. 19ra); "Baucia"
    (parsnip) "disposeth to lecchere" (f. 23vb); "Biscus" (mallow) "stireth
    to leccherie" (f. 31va); "Cinoglossa" (houndstongue) "is of might to
    norisch lecchere" (f. 62vb); "Iringus" (secacul) "encrese lecchere"
    (f. 104va); "Nasturcius" (cress) "Ete cocot encreseth lecchere" (f. 114vb);
    "Pastinaca" (also parsnip) "encreceth lecchere as almaundes do"
    (f. 119rb); etc. But for comparison, Henry Daniel describes many in-
    stances of herbs decreasing sexual desire: "Agnus Castus" (chaste tree)
    "refreyneth leccherie" and "qwencheth leccherie" (f. 8va); "Andrago"
    (purslane) "lesset streyng to leccherie" (f. 14va); "Benedicta" (hemlock)
    "stauncheth leccherie" (f. 26va); "Bisara" (rue) "fordoth leccherie"
    (f. 30rb); "Calamenta" (catnip) "distroyeth leccherie" (f. 41rb); "Cam-
    phora" is used "Ageyne lecchere" (f. 45va); "Cicoria" (chicory) is used
    "If fyr of lecchere take þe" (f. 61va); "Ciminus" (cumin) "lesseth lec-
    chere" (f. 61vb); etc.
41  Henry of Huntingdon, "Cicuta," *Anglicanus Ortus* #5.1.11, line 17
    (ed. and trans. Black), 282–3: "Et tu, Venus amans et amarus amor,
    superaris ..."
42  Henry of Huntingdon, "Nepta," *Anglicanus Ortus* #3.23, line 10 (ed. and
    trans. Black), 214–15: "Et stomachi morbis Bachi contrite liquore."

43  Henry of Huntingdon, "Pulegium," *Anglicanus Ortus* #2.16, lines 2–4 (ed. and trans. Black), 160:

O uirtus mira Tonantis,

Dans aliis alias persoluere mutua terras

Quo sit ut una domus sociandus partibus orbis!

44  Irma Taavitsainen, "Transferring classical discourse conventions into the vernacular," in *Medical and Scientific Writing in Late Medieval English*, ed. Irma Taavitsainen and Päivi Pahta (Cambridge: Cambridge University Press, 2004), 37–72: 67.

*Chapter Three*

Cᴏ

# Henry Daniel and His Medical Contemporaries in England

PETER MURRAY JONES

Contemporary authors do not feature in either the *Liber Uricrisiarum* or the herbal, and the most striking features of both these works are a creative engagement with earlier Latin authorities on the one hand, and observations drawn from Daniel's own experience or that of a few unnamed informants on the other. I will argue that, nevertheless, we can best appreciate what is novel and different about Daniel's work if we place it alongside the work of other English authors writing on medicine in the years between 1370 and 1425. By comparing his work with others in an extraordinary generation of medical writing in England, the idiosyncrasies of his approach and his relationship to contemporary understandings of medicine will emerge more clearly. Daniel owed little to his contemporaries in a direct fashion: he did not cite them or respond to their work. As one of the earliest of this generation of authors this is perhaps not so surprising in itself. But it seems that his project was different from theirs in important ways. It was different in terms of the readership he was trying to address, the language he used (English rather than Latin), and the aspects of medicine that most interested him. Despite these major differences in approach between Daniel and the others, some direct points of comparison do emerge once we look at Daniel's writing alongside that of other English authors like John Arderne, John Mirfield, John Bradmore, and Gilbert Kymer.[1] Daniel needs to be studied as a member of this extraordinary generation if his individuality is to be established, and just as important, if the points at which his work shares their preoccupations are to be identified.

The first part of this chapter will introduce these better-known English medical authors and briefly characterise their work in relation to that of Henry Daniel. The second part of the essay will foreground Henry Daniel as a Dominican, and assess his contributions by comparison with those of other contemporary friars who were compilers of medical writings or medical practitioners, or both. These other friars, Franciscan and Dominican, are much less well known than Daniel, and their writings circulated in smaller numbers of copies and in a more restricted cultural milieu. What is more, the style of compilation of these other mendicant works, emphasizing as it did the collective rather than the individual, was different to that of Daniel's *Liber Uricrisiarum* and his herbal treatise. And the other mendicant writings were in Latin rather than Middle English. Nevertheless, given that friars are usually simply left out of accounts of the development of medical writing and practice in England, it is important to examine the evidence we have in the writings of other mendicants. If Daniel was not the only friar writing on medicine, does that change the terms in which we judge his work?

The third and final part of the chapter will compare Daniel's herbal directly with that of a near contemporary work by a Franciscan friar, William Holme, entitled *De simplicibus medicinis*. This work too is devoted to medicinal simples, but offers a very different model of how to organise knowledge about herbs and other simples that will be useful to medical practitioners. The differences between the two works are the more striking since they rely on common sources of information about the natural substances they discuss. Henry Daniel's solution to the problem of advising the medical practitioner on simples emerges all the more clearly when the two works are compared directly.

### Henry Daniel and Contemporary Medical Authors

The best known of Daniel's contemporaries is surgeon and author John Arderne (1307–ca. 1380). His writings have survived in over fifty manuscript copies, and were widely admired at the time, and for a century after. Arderne wrote his treatise of fistula-in-ano in the 1370s, just when Daniel was assembling the *Liber Uricrisiarum*. Arderne's was the first and only medieval surgical treatise to focus at length on the conduct of one operation. Arderne also wrote a treatise on haemorrhoids, another on eye disease, a book of medicaments (*Liber medicinalium*), and a series of case histories of surgical treatment.[2] These works are all in Latin – despite Arderne's having been craft-trained as a surgeon, rather than university-educated. Surgeons in England are not generally assumed to be latinate. As a surgeon Arderne would not have been expected to be expert in uroscopy, which was the business of physicians, but there are several areas in which his work trod the same ground as that of Henry Daniel. For example, in the treatise on fistula-in-ano John Arderne includes a section on determining the right time for treatment. To operate on fistulae when the moon was in the signs of Scorpio, Libra, and Sagittarius was to risk grievous harm. Arderne incorporates a table with accompanying canon to enable the surgeon, equipped also with a calendar, to work out the moon's house on a given day.[3] The same table is found in the *Liber Uricrisiarum* Book 2 chapter 6 at the end of the long digression into planets and astronomy in Daniel's discussion of *lacteus* or milk-white colour of urine. Daniel's treatment of the matter is much longer and discusses many other astronomical topics, but both Arderne and Daniel introduce a table and instructions for finding the moon's house because of its immediate relevance to practical medicine and surgery.

This is not the only place where Arderne and Daniel cross paths. In Arderne's *Liber medicinalium* he interleaves a sequence of remedy-book recipes with descriptions of the medicinal virtues of different plants. These descriptions are similar to the much longer descriptions in Daniel's herbal, and sometimes make use of personal observations. In discussing juniper Arderne tells us about several places where it grows in abundance in southern England, including on Shooter's Hill in Kent on the road from London to Canterbury. Daniel draws attention to juniper flourishing in Kent, as well as near Shaftesbury in Dorset.[4]

A second English surgeon, John Bradmore, wrote his Latin *Philomena* ca. 1403–12. This is a lengthy treatise in seven parts, subdivided into *distinctiones* and chapters in scholastic mode, compiled from earlier Latin authorities on surgery (including Arderne), and interleaved with Bradmore's own cases and observations. These include his successful extraction of an arrowhead from the face of Prince Henry after the Battle of Shrewsbury in 1403.[5] This kind of case history, like those recorded by Arderne, is very much tied to claims of technical ingenuity on the part of the practitioner. Henry Daniel's case histories on the other hand are not personal claims to expertise.[6] Bradmore's writing in general, though, conforms much more closely than does Arderne to a scholastic model of organization. In fact, Bradmore may have copied the textual structure of the *Philomena* from John Mirfield (see below). The substance of the surgical teaching, the *doctrina*, is based firmly on the rational surgeries of authors like William of Saliceto[7] and Guy de Chauliac.[8] Other parts of the *Philomena* draw on John Mirfield as the mediating authority for earlier surgical writings, though Bradmore seldom acknowledges this debt. Guy de Chauliac is the principal source for Bradmore's text and is copied in many chapters almost word for word. Surgical authors, including William of Saliceto, Guy de Chauliac, Arderne, and Bradmore were all translated from Latin into Middle English before the middle of the fifteenth century.[9] There were sometimes substantial editorial interventions by the translators, but none of them attempted the kind of creative compilation that Daniel undertook with the materials for his *Liber Uricrisiarum*.

John Mirfield, a chaplain to St Bartholomew's Priory and Hospital in London, compiled two massive encyclopaedias in the 1390s. One, the *Florarium Bartholomei*, contains a section on the duties and etiquette of the physician, and gives guidance on when it is appropriate for the medical practitioner to give way to the priest at the bedside. But the other encyclopaedia, the *Breviarium Bartholomei,* is devoted entirely to medicine and surgery, and deals with ailments from head to foot, as well as covering fevers, compounding medicines, bloodletting, and a regimen of health.[10] Mirfield relies on a wide range of medical and surgical authorities but also records *experimenta* and charms that seem to derive from contemporary informants. Because the *Breviarium Bartholomei* is only known in full in two manuscripts, it is sometimes assumed that it can have been little known or used. This is quite wrong because Mirfield, as we have already seen in the case of his unacknowledged influence on John Bradmore, is one of the most quoted medical authorities in fifteenth-century England. He was also the only member of this group of writers contemporary with Daniel to write on uroscopy. The last *Distinctio* of the massive *Breviarium Bartholomei* was devoted to uroscopy. Incongruously it forms the last and tenth *Distinctio* of Part fifteen, a regimen of health, following immediately after a *Distinctio* on the use of cautery. Its appearance in this context as a relatively short section at the end of the *Breviarium Bartholomei* gives it the effect almost of an afterthought. Mirfield cites only one authority for this brief essay in diagnostics, Walter Agilon.[11] This very last chapter of the *Breviarium Bartholomei* consists of a short handy guide for the practitioner needing to make snap judgments on urines according to Agilon. The equivalent guide in the *Liber Uricrisiarum* is the "Rules of Isaac" at the very end of the beta version (not in the alpha version).[12] The *Liber Uricrisiarum* does not itself make much use of Agilon. But behind the six preceding chapters compiled by Mirfield on regions of urine, colours of urine, quality and quantity of urine, contents of urine, and sediment, it is clear that Mirfield shares with the *Liber Uricrisiarum* dependence on Isaac Israeli, *Liber de urinis*, and his commentators, even though this is never explicitly acknowledged in Mirfield's text.

By comparison with the surgeons Arderne and Bradmore, and John Mirfield, the chaplain to St Barthlomew's, university physicians do not make such a brave showing among English medical authors contemporary with Daniel. After John Gaddesden, writing at Oxford ca. 1313, the next university medical author of note is Simon Bredon. Bredon

(d. 1372), also of Merton College, Oxford, like Gaddesden, was DM by 1355, and seems to have left his *Trifolium* unfinished at this death. This late medical work was made possible by Simon Bredon's extraordinary collection of medical books, accompanied as it was by his own elaborately constructed indices and guides to the use of these books. What remains in one manuscript of the *Trifolium* is a fragment of what was planned as a massive compendium on medicine, but never finished; it is an intriguing (and unique) piece of evidence for the influence of the quantitative approach to assessing the impact of medicines originating at the University of Montpellier on English university medicine. Inevitably, as it was unfinished and never circulated, it was to have no impact on contemporary or later medical authors in England.[13]

The same might be said of the sole surviving work of Gilbert Kymer, physician to Duke Humfrey of Gloucester and later chancellor of the University of Oxford and dean of Salisbury. Kymer wrote a regimen of health for Duke Humfrey, the *Dietarium de sanitatis custodia*, in twenty-six chapters in 1424. It survives in one manuscript owned by William Botoner or Worcester (1415–ca. 1480), the antiquary with medical interests. It is more of an academic textbook on regimen and diet than a proper dietary for Duke Humfrey, though it does deal with a number of his personal afflictions in the last four chapters (when Kymer's own predilection for alchemical treatments also emerges). Kymer is supposed to have written a separate work on alchemy, which is not known to have survived. He seems to have shared this interest in alchemy put to medical use with several English friars, as we shall see, but not with Henry Daniel.[14]

These English medical authors make up an impressive group, particularly when compared with those flourishing in the periods before and after 1370–1425. Between John Gaddesden, whose *Rosa anglica* may be dated to ca. 1313, and John Arderne and Henry Daniel writing in the 1370s, there is little to note by way of original medical writing; the same might be said of the fifty years after 1425. There is one recently discovered exception, the *Tractatus phisice astronomice ad magnam securitatem exercitii artis medicine per solitudinem fratris Radulphi Hoby* of 1437.[15] Hoby's work of medical astrology was certainly written after Daniel's death but for our purposes what is most significant is that it was the work of a Franciscan friar. Linda Voigts brought Hoby's work to light, making him the second named English mendicant author on medicine after Daniel.[16]

There are no close parallels between Daniel's *Liber Uricrisiarum* and Hoby's *Tractatus phisice astronomice...* . Hoby frames his treatise around a series of medical questions that might be answered by astrological calculation (i.e., what may be the cause of the illness and the nature of the disease; whether or not the patient may be curable, and fourteen more). For this purpose he has no need to take account of Daniel's work on uroscopy. Hoby's work lies rather in the tradition of mendicant interest in astronomy and astrology manifested in the *Kalendarium* of John Somer, OFM, written in 1380. The *Kalendarium* was composed at the request of Thomas Kingsbury, the provincial minister of the Franciscans in England, for Joan of Kent (d. 1385), the mother of Richard II. A calendar with astronomical tables attached, it covered the four Metonic (nineteen-year) cycles for the period 1387 to 1462.[17] Hoby's treatise assumed ready access to such calendars and tables. Henry Daniel, writing before the calendar of John Somer, does cite the *Kalendarium* of the Cambridge-trained Walter Elveden, who was writing around 1350, to provide tables for the years 1330 to 1386. Later Elveden's almanac was continued forward by the Carmelite friar Nicholas of Lynn.[18]

We can see then that Henry Daniel belonged to a constellation of identifiable English writers on medicine between 1370 and 1425. These authors, particularly those in the surgical tradition, show awareness of other writers in their group. Thus Arderne is cited as an authority by both Mirfield and Bradmore. But Henry Daniel is not cited by any of them. There are a number of reasons why this should not surprise us. Henry Daniel was the only one of these authors to write in Middle English. He is self-conscious about this. He proclaims in the Prologue to the *Liber Uricrisiarum* that he has agreed to write his treatise in the vernacular language: "And also for Y haue noȝt mynde that I haue redde ne harde neyþer þis science giffen in English."[19] The *Liber Uricrisiarum* sets out to teach uroscopic diagnosis in painstaking detail for "I considerand meny men & diuerse þat couaiteþ to be experte of demyng of vrines" (Pro.42–3). He is seeking to establish a readership for these techniques of medical diagnosis beyond those educated at university and those brought up to read Latin. In this project Daniel aligns himself with a charitable impulse for translating Latin into Middle English, while being aware that making knowledge of uroscopy available to all and sundry runs the risk of that knowledge being exploited by those greedy for gold. Faye Getz has pointed out that Daniel and other later Dominicans like Thomas Moulton conceived of translation into English as a means by which the brothers could bring physic to the poor.[20] It is revealing to compare this mendicant approach to translation as a charitable obligation with that of John Arderne, who wrote in Latin. Arderne certainly wishes to equip his readers, imagined as fellow master surgeons, with the information and techniques they will need to perform complex surgical operations. He is happy to include many illustrations to supplement his text, though he suggests that certain operative procedures should be hidden from those who might try to copy them without understanding the necessary rationale. He uses Latin as his medium of address to his readers because he does not wish barber surgeons and empirics to be able to read and abuse his craft secrets. This did not prevent the translation of Arderne's own writings into Middle English early in the fifteenth century (the same fate befell Bradmore's *Philomena*).[21]

Henry Daniel's *Liber Uricrisiarum* was the only medical treatise amongst this late medieval group to be written in Middle English, but it was also the only one devoted primarily to knowledge of uroscopy. The other treatises in the group of English medical authors were contributions to surgery, or to therapeutics through compound medicines and regimen, subjects that the *Liber Uricrisiarum* deliberately eschewed. Despite this comparatively small area of overlap between Henry Daniel's *Liber Uricrisiarum* and the other English writers on medicine, what is more remarkable is that such an essential part of the practice of physic should be so neglected by authors other than Henry Daniel. Given that uroscopy was the central part of the art of diagnosis for a medieval physician, and that medieval physicians set themselves apart from other practitioners by their ability to diagnose on rational principles, why should the other writers in the group have by and large neglected uroscopy? This is far from an easy question to answer with confidence, in the absence of evidence from the authors themselves. The most prominent authors in this generation were not university teachers, and so not required to teach or comment on uroscopy (but that of course applies to Daniel too). Nor in fact was there a flourishing original literature on uroscopy in Europe after 1200 even at the great continental universities, although there were learned commentaries on the older writings. There was instead an efflorescence in England and elsewhere of short prescriptive guides to uroscopy in Latin and the vernacular circulating in the late fourteenth and fifteenth centuries, presumably targeted at medical practitioners.[22] Henry Daniel was exceptional, not just in writing about uroscopy in Middle English, but in taking such trouble to collate different Latin authorities and attempting to systematise them into a comprehensive manual on the subject.

### Henry Daniel and Medicine of the Friars

So far I have considered Henry Daniel's *Liber Uricrisiarum* as one of a group of medical treatises authored in England ca. 1370–1425, and looked for points of similarity or difference between Daniel's work and the others in the group. But there is another medical treatise that can be compared directly with the *Liber Uricrisiarum*, not least because it was compiled by English friars. This is the *Tabula medicine*, which survives in three complete manuscripts from the fifteenth century, and whose colophon in one manuscript declares that it was compiled between 1416 and 1425.[23] It refers by name to a number of English friars, Franciscans and Dominicans, contemporaries or figures within living memory of the compilers (but does not refer to Henry Daniel). Those mentioned in the *Tabula medicine* were either authors or practitioners of medicine – sometimes it is not possible to tell one from the other. The text itself is organised as an encyclopaedic handbook of medicine, and it was compiled by accumulating remedies within spaces left in an original manuscript under each disease heading. The ordering of these headings is alphabetical, a form favoured by mendicant authors in all fields of learning. One later writer thought that the compilers were Franciscans. Thomas Fayreford, who practised medicine in the West Country in the second quarter of the fifteenth century, identified the *Tabula medicine* as a work compiled by Franciscans ("ut dicunt fratres minores") in his medical commonplace book.[24]

From which authorities was the *Tabula medicine* compiled? The works that are quoted are well-known medieval sources for practical medicine. More than twenty-five different sources are used, and there are the expected citations of the great medical authorities, Hippocrates, Galen, Avicenna, and Rasis, as well as works on surgery, materia medica, and encyclopaedias – in the latter field, most often cited was Bartholomaeus Anglicus (OFM), *De proprietatibus rerum*.[25] Often these citations are vague as to which text in particular is being cited, giving only a name. But the most frequently cited authorities over the *Tabula medicine* as a whole, as might be anticipated in an English work in therapeutics of this period, are Gilbertus Anglicus, Bernard de Gordon, John Gaddesden, and John Arderne. Less easily anticipated is the use of the *Breviarium Bartholomei* of John Mirfield, as discussed in the previous section of this chapter. As chaplain at the Priory and Hospital of St Bartholomew's in Smithfield, in London, he must have been a contemporary or near contemporary of the compilers of the *Tabula medicine*. It seems that the original compilers of the *Tabula medicine* were simply using the materials most readily at hand in England for anyone interested in compiling an encyclopaedic remedy book. The compilers were looking to add remedies for the chosen disease headings that could be copied from authors of authoritative texts on practical medicine. But alongside these written sources were remedies attributed to, or tested by, particular named friars.

If the *Tabula medicine* was compiled by Franciscans, as Thomas Fayreford thought, it did not refer exclusively to members of that order. Dominicans are mentioned in the text too, most notably Geoffrey Launde (or Laud, as the text has it), who is credited with a number of remedies. He was licensed by the General of his Order to act as confessor to Edmund, Duke of Aumale (from 1402 Duke of York), in 1398 and to practise medicine within the Duke's household or elsewhere.[26] Amongst the Franciscan friars named as sources for remedies, or for having tested their efficacy, William Holme is mentioned more than one hundred times in the course of the text. He treated a number of patients named in the *Tabula medicine*, including the Franciscan Provincial Minister Nicholas Fakenham, members of the Warwickshire-based Trussell family, and the afore-mentioned Duke. Holme was also the author of two medical texts. One is the *De simplicibus medicinis*, which I will compare below with Henry Daniel's herbal. The other is a much shorter *Tractatus de medicinis*, found so far only in Cambridge, Trinity College MS O.9.10, f. 114–19. It is a kind of medical *Practica*, gathering remedies in roughly head to toe order, but as it moves down from the head the remedies became fewer and shorter, as if the work in progress tailed away before finishing incomplete. Another Franciscan mentioned in the *Tabula medicine* as an authority for several remedies is William Appleton or Appulton, retained for life in 1373 by John of Gaunt as his "phisicien et surgien," and killed in the Peasants' Revolt of 1381. Appleton may also be the Franciscan friar mentioned by Arderne as his only rival in the surgical operation for fistula-in-ano, although there were other friars with surgical expertise.[27]

This wealth of citation of friars as authors and practitioners in the *Tabula Medicine* is in marked contrast to the *Liber Uricrisiarum*. The few case histories in Daniel's work do not refer to friar practitioners of medicine, and the authorities cited do not include mendicant authors (the beta version does however mention Bartholomaeus Anglicus, author of *De proprietatibus rerum*). Taking the *Tabula medicine* into account helps us to repopulate late medieval England with friars as both medical practitioners and authors, whereas the *Liber Uricrisiarum* on its own might suggest that Henry Daniel was the only mendicant with medical interests. Further, the *Tabula medicine* suggests that the Dominicans and Franciscan orders both supplied brethren who practised medicine. The compilers wanted their readers to profit from the experience of practitioners in both orders.

John Arderne's writings help to confirm this impression left by the *Tabula medicine* of the visibility in Henry Daniel's time of friars as medical practitioners. In one of his case histories Arderne refers to a

Franciscan as an expert on wound treatment, whose remedy for *malum mortuum* he describes. It had excellent results for the patient and was subsequently tested successfully by Arderne himself.[28] In another case Arderne refers to a friar as his informant on a particular course of treatment, and as we have already seen, Arderne thought of a Franciscan (perhaps William Appleton) as his only rival in performing the complex and dangerous operation for fistula-in-ano.

Not all the friars identified by name in the *Tabula medicine* were medical practitioners. One friar who is mentioned under fifteen different disease headings in the *Tabula medicine* is Robert Wainflet. He seems to be otherwise unknown as an author but within the *Tabula medicine* he is deferred to as an authority on the theoretical understanding of illness. For example, under the heading "Caput" [Head], the text describes the three cells of the brain, the homes of imagination, rationality, and memory. Each cell has its own complexional balance. Damage to any cell causes distinctive patterns of mental disturbance. Wainflet's views resemble those expressed by William of Conches, drawing on the *Pantegni* of Constantinus Africanus, and repeated in the thirteenth century by Vincent of Beauvais OP in his *Speculum naturale*.[29] A longer account of the cells of the brain, their complexions, and functions is to be found in the *Liber Uricrisiarum*, in Book 2 chapter 7 under the colour "karope." As with the section on the planets and astronomy discussed earlier, this section on brain anatomy is inserted wholesale into the text of this chapter abruptly. The justification for including it is the well-known proposition in uroscopy that the regions of the body (including the head and brain) have corresponding regions in the urine glass (so that the *circulus* corresponds to the head).[30] Amidst the discussion of the four regions, we find a description of the cells of the brain and their functions, corresponding to that in Wainflet. Further, the same ailments that hinder brain function in the passage from Wainflet are also described by Daniel in Book 3 chapter 2 on the *circulus* in urine. The passages in the two works, however, are quite different in scale and purpose. In the *Tabula medicine* the abbreviated quotation from Wainflet serves as a kind of cross-reference to the diseases of the head mentioned elsewhere in the text under different headings ("Epilepsia," "Mania," "Frenesis," and "Litargia"). Henry Daniel by contrast translates and compiles his text on the cells of the brain so that it will provide an anatomical key to the discussion of diagnosis by analysis of regions of the urine glass in Book 3 of the *Liber Uricrisiarum*.

Uncovering the citations of the otherwise unknown Robert Wainflet in the *Tabula medicine* suggests that Henry Daniel may not have been the only mendicant author who dealt with theoretical medical topics.

The brief glimpse of Wainflet is tantalizing because direct sources for medical learning amongst the friars are so hard to find. Here we are handicapped by what has been lost with the Reformation in England. The disappearance of almost all of the medical books that must once have been held in mendicant libraries, and the lack of surviving archives for the convents and provinces of the friars, make it only too likely that we have lost sight of significant contributions to medical learning made by the friars.[31]

Mendicants in England would have been far more visible to their contemporaries as authors and practitioners of medicine than they are to us today. This is one thing we can learn from close reading of the *Tabula medicine*. But there are also suggestive points of comparison between the *Tabula medicine* and the *Liber Uricrisiarum*. I am going to single out just one of these here, the use of *experimenta*. Friar Robert Wainflet, whose consideration on the anatomy of the brain we have just met, also emerges in the *Tabula medicine* as a keen exponent of their usefulness. One kind of *experimenta* is prognostic tests designed to forecast the outcomes of illnesses or the success of treatment (other medical authorities use the term *experimenta* in a wider sense).[32] Under the heading "Lepra" there are four such *experimenta*: for example, take a newly hatched egg, put it in the client's urine, wait for an hour and break the egg – if the egg is corrupt he is incurable, if it is still sweet he can be cured. Two of these *experimenta* for "Lepra" are credited to Robert Wainflet. Five *experimenta* are found as prognostics under the heading "Infirmus" (the sick person). These are tests to determine whether the patient will live or die, useful both to determine whether to treat a patient and to forecast the outcome of the illness, treated or untreated. One is called *proba vite* or "test of life," and suggests taking bear's gall, cooking it with white gum arabic to make a plaster, and then putting it over the area of the liver for nine days. If the plaster stays on for this time, the patient will live; if not, he dies. These *experimenta* are found not only in the *Tabula medicine* but also in the works of other late fourteenth-century authors like John Arderne and John Mirfield.

They are also to be found in the *Liber Uricrisiarum*. In Book 2 chapter 3 Daniel deals with the diagnosis of phthisis, and he mentions two *experimenta* that may be employed. The first suggests the spittle of the patient should be heated over a fire or in the coals, and if it smells foul, it indicates phthisis. If the patient is losing hair too he is likely to die from it. The question of whether the patient will live can also be tested by seeing if his spittle floats in the dish of water: floating augurs well, sinking badly (2.3.451–79). Two more such *experimenta* are used by Daniel in relation to conception. He introduces them by saying: "Now for to

knowen & weten when woman hath conceyuede & when noght, auctoures techen meny expermentez" (3.16.238–9). Before discussing the
two experiments Daniel sets out the signs of pregnancy as generally
agreed among medical authors. The first of his *experimenta* is taken from
Hippocrates and involves giving the woman *mellicratum* to drink and
seeing if she feels pain. The second *experimentum* is to establish whose
fault it is in a couple that the woman cannot conceive, and is taken from
the *Trotula*. The man and the woman piss in different pots of bran; the
pots are left for a week or two and the party at fault will be known by
the presence of worms and a foul stink (3.16.362–9).[33] While Daniel is
happy to encourage the use of these *experimenta* for fertility, he is cau-
tious elsewhere in the *Liber Uricrisiarum* about the use of urine to identify the father of a child, or to predict the sex or colour of a calf. He hits
out at those swindlers who pretend to be able to tell more from urine
than is authorised by true learning, the "vnwise leches – þat in þise
dayes ar callede dogg-leches os þise entremetoures & þise bolde braggers þat stonde in chateryng & in clatering & noght in connyng, and þat
onely for mony wynnyng" (2.12.59–62). This worry also emerges in the
Latin verse epilogue to the entire *Liber Uricrisiarum*. After some lines
devoted to the usual topoi of apology for what is missing or wrong in
the text and the hope that more learned readers will correct mistakes,
he launches suddenly into an attack on those who claim to be able to
tell whether a foetus is the offspring of a priest or a soldier, or whether
a calf will be black, red, or spotted.[34]

It may seem surprising that any friar should even find it proper to
discuss such matters as *experimenta* for conception. But Henry Daniel
was not alone in an avid interest in matters of generation. One manuscript of the *Tabula medicine* has been annotated by a reader in Latin:
"for woman look at these headings": "Aborsus," "Conceptio," "Fetus,"
"Impregnatio," "Matrix," "Menstrua," "Mulier," "Partus," "Pregnans,"
"Puer," "Secundina," "Vulva," and "Sterilitas."[35] Under these headings there are many references to friars as authorities on medicines for
human reproduction, including William Holme and Geoffrey Launde,
whom we have met already. At the end of the heading "Sterilitas" in the
*Tabula medicine* there are five tests for telling whether sterility is the fault
of the woman or the man. One involves giving the woman a subfumigation through her sexual organs and is attributed to Hippocrates.[36]
The last one in the series suggests that the woman should be given a
drop of balsam mixed with warm water on a pad, which is then put
into the vagina attached to a thread. If the womb takes it in then the
woman can conceive; if not, not. This test is attributed to John Gaddesden. In fact both the Hippocratic subfumigation and the balsam test are

in the chapter on sterility in the *Rosa anglica*, and the compilers of the *Tabula medicine* probably took both directly from that source.[37] They do not express any worries about "dog-leeches," who claimed expertise in foretelling the outcome of pregnancies.

## Daniel's Herbal and Holme's *De simplicibus medicinis*

By contrast with the many surviving copies of the *Liber Uricrisiarum*, Henry Daniel's herbal is known only in two manuscripts in the British Library, one of them evidently only about half finished. The two manuscripts differ in that Additional MS 27329, which is complete, has two series of entries, one for herbs and one for other medicinal simples, both alphabetically ordered. By contrast Arundel MS 42 has only one series of entries, running only from A to G, and interfiles the herbs with other kinds of medicinal simple. It is not clear yet which of these versions was made first, or whether one represents second thoughts about organization by the compiler, Henry Daniel himself. Both versions refer back to the *Liber Uricrisiarum*, so the herbal is clearly the later work. As noted on the herbal page of the Henry Daniel project website, entries in both manuscripts commonly include information on synonyms for names of plants, occasional etymologies, complexional qualities (hot/cold, wet/dry and in what degree), the appearance of the plant, what the plant or other ingredient is medically good for, recipes for specific medicines, and information on where particular plants grow or can be obtained and what light Daniel's personal experience can shed on their use. As in the case of the *Liber Uricrisiarum*, the herbal is a compilation from different sources, and some of the learned authorities cited are not based on original writings but on more recent sources, unacknowledged, from which the learned citations come.[38]

William Holme's *De simplicibus medicinis* makes an interesting comparison with Daniel's herbal. Unlike the herbal it is a Latin text. The explicit to the long text reads in translation: "here ends the best treatise on simple medicines for particular sicknesses of the body, by brother William Holme 'medicus' of the order of friars minor about the year of our Lord 1415, excerpted from 12 doctors of medicine [their names follow] and others, compiled excellently into alphabetical order, first of simple medicines and then of the particular illnesses."[39] This text is known in two manuscripts, one of which was written in Oxford in 1435 by William Bedmyster, Fellow of New College.[40] The second manuscript dates from towards the end of the fifteenth century, and was owned by Thomas Deynman (d. 1501), "medicus" and Fellow, later Master, of Peterhouse, Cambridge.[41] So instead of a putatively Franciscan scribe and context, as with the *Tabula medicine*, we have a text known to us only through university men. The method of compilation of *De simplicibus medicinis* is straightforward in plan, but must have presented considerable problems to Holme in execution. The alphabetical headings of illnesses encountered by the reader (i.e., the result of the second exercise in alphabetization mentioned in the explicit) are quite similar to those used in the *Tabula medicine*. Since the *Tabula medicine* was compiled after *De simplicibus medicinis*, it may have been influenced by Holme's method rather than vice versa. But none of the content of *De simplicibus medicinis* is repeated in the *Tabula medicine*.

There are 214 headings for illnesses in *De simplicibus medicinis*, though some of the headings, strictly speaking, refer not to illnesses but to things that medicines can do. Thus there is a heading for "Atrahere" that deals with drawing out to the surface things (like thorns) that have been absorbed into the body. "Aqua citrina" refers to a fluid that needs to be expelled, and the entry ends with a cross reference to "Ydropisis" (dropsy). Similarly, "Humor" means humours that needs to be purged, although is not itself an illness. Other headings deal with parts of the body like "Auris" (ear) and "Lingua" (tongue), that stand for the illnesses that may afflict these parts. Under each heading there is an alphabetical list of the medicinal simples that are effective in treating that illness. These appear as subheadings and the number of them varies from as few as five, in the very first entry "Abhominatio," to more than a hundred ("Stomacus"). The work of drawing this material out of the authors he read, and organizing it under these headings in two sequences each in alphabetical order, must have been laborious and complicated, and Holme would have had to create some kind of file system. While the *De simplicibus medicinis* is the only medical work of this kind compiled in England, it employs the same kind of method as do study aids for biblical and theological students compiled by Franciscans.[42] The purpose was to save the labour of searching through numbers of authoritative texts to find the passages required to insert in a sermon or homily on a particular subject. Holme's readers would have been able to use *De simplicibus medicinis* to see at a glance the different remedial options available when faced with a particular illness.

At the end of each entry for a simple to be used in treating an illness Holme gives the name of the authority from which his information is drawn. The list of authors in the explicit to the text is as follows: Avicenna, Almasor, Bartholomeus, Constantinus, Gerardus, Macer, Mesue, Petrus perybonensis, Platearius, Serapion, Willelmus de placencia, and Ysaac, and others.[43] They represent the leading authorities on the use of simple medicines, some being Islamicate authors translated into Latin, but others Western authors like the Salernitan Matthaeus Platearius, Odo de Meung (Macer) writing in verse, the Franciscan encyclopaedist Bartholomaeus Anglicus, or scholastics like Gerard of Berry and the surgeon William of Saliceto. After each entry for a simple used to treat a particular disease in *De simplicibus medicinis* William Holme gives the name of the authority from which he derives this information. I have checked his citations from all the authors listed and they are carefully and accurately transcribed from the source texts. They do not represent the most recent writers on medicine but those whose works were in circulation around 1300, a century before Holme compiled his text. The most unusual name found in the list of authorities is the hardest to identify from the name given. Petrus Hispanus was known to Holme and to the compilers of the *Tabula medicine* as Petrus Perybonensis, a name not found elsewhere to my knowledge. But his *Thesaurus pauperum* is a well-known thirteenth-century handbook of compound medicines, claimed to be for the use of those unable to afford expensive drugs. Its appearance in *De simplicibus medicinis* is anomalous because the *Thesaurus pauperum* is not a list of medicinal simples and their uses, like the other authorities. Accordingly, whereas the shortest entries in Holme's text indicate only that a certain simple works in a case of a particular illness, those taken from Petrus Hispanus are more discursive and suggest the combining of simples to make compound medicines.

Daniel's herbal draws from many of the same sources as does Holme: *Circa instans* (Platearius), Bartholomeus Anglicus, Macer, Avicenna, Rasis, ps-Mesue, Serapion, and the *Pantegni* of Constantine, but casts its net much wider than the twelve authorities identified by Holme. Thus Daniel uses extensively the *Anglicanus ortus* of Henry of Huntingdon,[44] the anonymous *Alphita*,[45] the *Antidotarium Nicholai*,[46] the *Natural History* of Pliny the Elder, and the experiments of the *Liber vaccae*, attributed by Daniel to Plato.[47] And Daniel does not confine himself to the listing of medicinal uses of simples for particular illnesses, as the website description of the herbal makes clear. His approach is discursive and descriptive, going to considerable trouble to distinguish different varieties of an herb, the uses of various parts of the herb, and features that might enable the reader to find it and be certain of its identification. Sometimes Daniel gives complete recipes for the treatment of an illness, with an indication of quantities and method of preparation, not just the principal ingredient, as found in *De simplicibus medicinis* (such detailed recipes are of course characteristic, however, of the *Tabula medicine*). Daniel often refers to opinions held by undocumented sources "some say ..." or to the practices of "conyng folk" (see the entry for

"Arnoglossa"). Under "Apolinaris" (or mandrake) Daniel tells us that he was in the company of three men who wished to establish whether a man who carried a mandrake on his person would always be flush with money; the party examined the bundle carried by such a man in his absence, but found only a single penny along with the mandrake root.

## Conclusion

Henry Daniel's ambitions to write encyclopaedic handbooks of uroscopy and of the knowledge of medicinal simples were shared with contemporary medical writers. John Arderne's works considered as a whole aim to do much the same for surgery and for several branches of practical medicine (for instance purgation and ophthalmology). John Mirfield's enormous *Breviarium Bartholomei* embraced practical medicine, surgery, regimen, and even uroscopy. The intended audience for these works seems to have been readers who were health consumers or practitioners in diagnosis, therapeutics, and regimen rather than scholastic academics. These works were meant to appeal to those who wanted practical guidance on health matters, not those working in university milieux. Simon Bredon and Gilbert Kymer on the other hand seem to have been more concerned with exhibiting their scholastic credentials and showing how up to date they were with medical learning. John Bradmore falls somewhere in the middle of this spectrum, modelling his work on compendious scholastic surgeries, but salting his text with case histories and personal observations. Henry Daniel stands out from the other medical encyclopaedists in choosing first to concentrate on uroscopy, but his predilection for venturing into byways not strictly necessary to his central theme meant that he sometimes found himself in territory also explored by his contemporaries (calendar astrology, use of *experimenta*, and brain function and disorders are the examples we have examined).

Other friars practising or writing medicine do not feature in Henry Daniel's works, nor his in theirs. As a Dominican he may not have known the Franciscans later involved in compiling the *Tabula medicine*, or those described there as practising medicine. Yet friar practitioners do surface in contemporary sources. John Arderne talks about Franciscan practitioners as competitors and sources of remedies, so we know that they were visible in the medical marketplace. Daniel is the first mendicant author on medicine whose works survive to us; William Holme, Ralph Hoby, and Friar Narborough came later. But the only text identified so far that gives us insight into a distinctively mendicant knowledge and practice of medicine is the *Tabula medicine* of 1416–25.

The most obvious difference between Henry Daniel and contemporary medical authors, whether mendicants or not, was his choice of language. By committing himself to the project of charitable translation he set out to make his knowledge of the principles of uroscopy and of medicinal simples available in English. Other works aimed at medical practitioners preferred to stick with Latin and must have had good reason to suppose that Latin could be read by their target audience (including friars of course). But it was more than simply a matter of who could read what. As we have seen from a direct comparison between Holme's *De simplicibus medicinis* and Daniel's herbal, the latter was aiming to do more than provide a streamlined tool for accessing a range of authorities on the use of medicinal simples. As editorial work on the herbal advances, the originality of Henry Daniel's approach in this work will come into sharper focus.[48]

## NOTES

1  The English medical authors and practitioners mentioned in this chapter will usually have entries in the following reference works: Richard Sharpe, *A Handlist of the Latin Writers of Great Britain and Ireland before 1540* (Turnhout: Brepols, 1997); *ODNB*; Charles H. Talbot and E.A. Hammond, *The Medical Practitioners in Medieval England: A Biographical Register* (London: Wellcome Historical Medical Library, 1965); Faye Marie Getz, "Medieval Practitioners in Medieval England." *Social History of Medicine* 3 (1990): 245–83. I should like to thank Sarah Star and M. Teresa Tavormina for their great help with this chapter.

2  Peter Murray Jones, "John Arderne and the Mediterranean Tradition of Scholastic Surgery," in *Practical Medicine from Salerno to the Black Death*, ed. Luis Garcia-Ballester, Roger French, Jon Arrizabalaga and Andrew Cunningham (Cambridge: Cambridge University Press, 1994), 289–321.

3  Arderne, *Treatises of Fistula in Ano, Hæmorrhoids, and Clysters*, ed. D'Arcy Power (London: Oxford University Press, 1910), 16–19.

4  Arderne: Glasgow University Library, Hunter MS 112, f. 16r; Daniel: "Amifructus juniperi" in the herbal.

5  See Sheila J. Lang, "John Bradmore and his book *Philomena*." *Social History of Medicine* 5 (1992): 121–30; Lang, "John Bradmore and the Case of the Bitten Man: A Tantalising Link between Three Medieval Surgical Manuscripts." *Social History of Medicine* (2020), hkaa014, https://doi.org/10.1093/shm/hkaa014; and Theodore R. Beck, *The Cutting Edge: Early History of the Surgeons of London* (London: Lund Humphries, 1974), 55–6.

6   For more on Daniel's case histories, see Hannah Bower's chapter in this volume, "'Her ovn self seid me': The Function of Anecdote in Henry Daniel's *Liber Uricrisiarum*," 133–57.

7   Jole Agrimi and Chiara Crisciani, "The Science and Practice of Medicine in the Thirteenth Century According to Guglielmo da Saliceto, Italian Surgeon," in *Practical Medicine from Salerno to the Black Death*, ed. Luis Garcia-Ballester, Roger French, Jon Arrizabalaga, and Andrew Cunningham (Cambridge: Cambridge University Press, 1994), 60–87.

8   Guy de Chauliac, *Inventarium sive Chirurgia Magna*, edited by Michael R. McVaugh (Leiden: E.J. Brill, 1997); McVaugh, *The Rational Surgery of the Middle Ages* (Florence: SISMEL/Edizioni del Galluzzo, 2006).

9   Linda Ehrsam Voigts, "Scientific and Medical Books," in *Book Production and Publishing in Britain, 1375–1475*, ed. Jeremy Griffiths and Derek Pearsall (Cambridge: Cambridge University Press, 1989), 345–402; George Keiser, ed. *A Manual of the Writings in Middle English 1050–1500*, Vol. 10 *Works of Science and Information* (New Haven: Connecticut Academy of Arts and Sciences, 1998); *eVK2* 2014.

10   Percival Horton-Smith Hartley and Harold Richard Aldridge, *Johannes de Mirfeld of St Bartholomew's, Smithfield: His Life and Works* (Cambridge: Cambridge University Press, 1936); Getz, "John Mirfield and the Breviarium Bartholomei: The Medical Writings of a Clerk at St Bartholomew's Hospital in the Later Fourteenth Century," *Society for the Social History of Medicine Bulletin* 37 (1985): 24–6.

11   *Gualteri Agilonis Summa medicinalis*. Studien zur Geschichte der Medizin Beiheft 3, ed. Paul Diepgen (Leipzig: Johann Ambrosius Barth, 1911).

12   For a detailed account of how contents of the text vary across its different versions, see E. Ruth Harvey's chapter in this volume, "Textual Layers in the *Liber Uricrisiarum*," 87–107.

13   Talbot, "Simon Bredon (c.1300–1372), Physician, Mathematician, and Astronomer," *British Journal for the History of Science* 1 (1962–3): 19–30; Faye Marie Getz, "The Faculty of Medicine before 1500," in *The History of the University of Oxford*, vol. 2, *Late Medieval Oxford*, ed. J.I. Catto and T.A.R. Evans (Oxford: Oxford University Press, 1992), 400–4; Getz, *Medicine in the English Middle Ages* (Princeton, NJ: Princeton University Press, 1998).

14   Glenn James Hardingham, "The Regimen in Late Medieval England." PhD diss., University of Cambridge, 2005, ch. 2; London, British Library, Sloane MS 4, ff. 63–102v.

15   M. Teresa Tavormina, in "The Heirs of Henry Daniel," 108–32, deals with Daniel's Franciscan editor and imitator, Friar Narborough, writing ca. 1450.

16   Linda Ehrsam Voigts, "Wolfenbüttel HAB Cod. Guelf. 51. 9. Aug. 4° and BL, Harley MS. 3542: Complementary Witnesses to Ralph Hoby's 1437

Treatise on Astronomical Medicine." *Electronic British Library Journal* (2008), Article 10; Voigts, "The Medical Astrology of Ralph Hoby, Fifteenth Century Franciscan," in *The Friars in Medieval Britain: Proceedings of the 2007 Harlaxton Symposium*, ed. Nicholas Rogers (Donington: Shaun Tyas, 2010), 152–68.

17  *The Kalendarium of John Somer*, ed. Linne R. Mooney (Athens, GA: University of Georgia Press, 1998).

18  John North, *Chaucer's Universe* (Oxford, Clarendon Press, 1988), ch. 3.

19  *Liber Uricrisiarum: A Reading Edition*, edited by E. Ruth Harvey, M. Teresa Tavormina, and Sarah Star (University of Toronto Press, 2020), Pro.12–13. Subsequent quotations from the edition are cited parenthetically by book, chapter, and line number. The Prologue is cited by line number. This issue is pursued further in Sarah Star's chapter in this volume, "The 'almost-Latin' Medical Language of Late Medieval England," 158–74.

20  Getz, "Charity, Translation, and the Language of Medical Learning in Medieval England." *Bulletin of the History of Medicine* 64 (1999): 1–17.

21  Jones, "John Arderne and the Mediterranean Tradition of Scholastic Surgery" (1994), 289–321; Jones, "Language and Register in English Medieval Surgery," in *Language in Medieval Britain: Networks and Exchanges: Proceedings of the 2013 Harlaxton Symposium*, ed. Mary Carruthers (Donington: Shaun Tyas, 2015), 74–89.

22  Tavormina, "Uroscopy in Middle English: A Guide to the Texts and Manuscripts," *Studies in Medieval & Renaissance History*. 3rd series. 11 (2014): 1–154; *eTK* 2017 (subject search: urine and uroscopy).

23  Jones, "The *'Tabula medicine'*: An Evolving Encyclopedia," in *English Manuscript Studies, 1100–1700*, volume 14, *Regional Manuscripts, 1200–1700*, ed. A.S.G. Edwards (London: British Library, 2008), 60–85; Jones, "Mediating Collective Experience: The *Tabula Medicine* (1416–1425) as a Handbook for Medical Practice," in *Between Text and Patient: The Medical Enterprise in Medieval and Early Modern Europe*, Micrologus' Library 39, ed. Florence Eliza Glaze and Brian K. Nance (Florence: SISMEL/Edizioni del Galluzzo, 2011), 279–307.

24  London, British Library, Harley MS 2558, f. 148v; Jones, "Harley MS 2558: A Fifteenth-Century Medical Commonplace Book," in *Manuscript Sources of Medieval Medicine: A Book of Essays*, ed. Margaret R. Schleissner (New York, London: Garland, 1995), 35–54; Jones, "Thomas Fayreford: An English Fifteenth-Century Medical Practitioner," in *Medicine from the Black Death to the French Disease*, ed. Roger French, Jon Arrizabalaga, Andrew Cunningham and Luis Garcia-Ballester (Aldershot: Ashgate, 1998), 156–83.

25  Heinz Meyer, *Die Enzyklopädie des Bartholomäus Anglicus. Untersuchungen zur Überlieferungs- und Rezeptionsgeschichte von 'De proprietatibus rerum'*

(Munich: Wilhelm Fink, 2000); *Bartholomaeus Anglicus De Proprietatibus Rerum*, Vol. 6 Liber XVII, ed. Iolanda Ventura (Turnhout: Brepols, 2007).

26 Jones, "Mediating Collective Experience" (2011), 285.

27 Richard Firth Green, "Friar William Appleton and the Date of Langland's B Text." *The Yearbook of Langland Studies* 11 (1997): 87–96.

28 London, British Library, Sloane MS 56, f. 90r.

29 Italo Ronca, *Guillelmi de Conchis Dragmaticon philosophiae* (Turnhout: Brepols, 1997), 239–43; Ynez Violé O'Neill, "William of Conches' Descriptions of the Brain," *Clio Medica* 3 (1968): 203–23.

30 Cambridge, University Library, MS Gg.3.29, f. 88r. Joanne Jasin, "The Transmission of Learned Medical Literature in the Middle English *Liber Uricrisiarum*," *Medical History* 37 (1993): 313–29.

31 Kenneth William Humphreys, *The Friars' Libraries*. Corpus of British Medieval Library Catalogues 1 (London: British Library in association with the British Academy, 1990), xv–xxii; *Medieval Libraries of Great Britain 3* (*MLGB3*), 2015.

32 Michael R. McVaugh, "The Experimenta of Arnald of Villanova," *Journal of Medieval and Renaissance Studies* 1 (1971): 107–18; Jole Agrimi and Chiara Crisciani, "Per una ricerca su 'Experimentum-experimenta': riflessione epistemological e tradizione medica (secoli XIII–XV)," in *Presenza del lessico greco e latino nelle lingue contemporanee: ciclo di lezioni tenute all'Universita do Macerate nell'a.a. 1987–88*, ed. Pietro Janni and Innocenzo Mazzini (Macerata: Universita di Macerata, 1990), 9–49.

33 Cf. *The Trotula: A Medieval Compendium of Women's Medicine*, edited by Monica H. Green (Philadelphia, PA: University of Pennsylvania Press, 2001), 94–5, which provides an edition of the *Trotula*, the most important medieval collection of material on women's ailments. This test is also found in book 2 cap 3 of the *Liber Uricrisiarum*. See also London, British Library, Harley MS 2558 f.168v for similar generation *experimenta*.

34 Cambridge, University Library, MS Gg.3.29, f. 169r.

35 London, University College, MS Lat 11, f. 2*v (Jones, "Mediating Collective Experience" [2011], 302).

36 Two of these *experimenta* in fact are found originally in Hippocrates, *Aphorisms*, 5.11–12.

37 Gaddesden, *Rosa Anglica Practica Medicinae* (Pavia: Fransiscus Girardengus and Johannes Antonius Birreta, 1492), f. 95v.

38 For instance one such intermediate authority is a writer called by Daniel "*Auctor bolus*, whos name Y fynde no3t" (British Library, Arundel MS 42, f. 5v). *Auctor bolus* cites a number of Greco-Arabic sources, incl. Dioscorides, Avicenna, Serapion, Galen, Averroes, Constantine, Mesue, et al. See https://henrydaniel.utoronto.ca/herbal/sources/.

39   Rodney M. Thomson, *A Descriptive Catalogue of the Medieval Manuscripts in the Library of Peterhouse, Cambridge* (Cambridge: D.S. Brewer, 2016), 99.

40   A.B. Emden, *A Biographical Register of the University of Oxford to A.D. 1500* (Oxford: Clarendon Press, 1957), 1: 147.

41   *ODNB.*

42   Mary A. Rouse and Richard H. Rouse, *Authentic Witnesses: Approaches to Medieval Texts and Manuscripts* (Notre Dame IN: University of Notre Dame Press, 1991), 221–55.

43   The works referred to are as follows: Avicenna, *Liber canonis*, bk 2 *De simplicibus medicine; Liber Rasis ad almansorem*, bk 3; Bartholomaeus Anglicus, *De proprietatibus rerum*, bk 17; Constantine the African, *Pantegni, Practica* bk 2; Gerardus Bituricensis, *Glossae super viaticum Constantini Africani;* Macer, *De viribus herbarum;* ps-Mesue, *De simplicibus medicine;* Petrus Hispanus, *Thesaurus pauperum;* Mattheus Platearius, *Circa instans; Liber Serapionis agregatus in medicinis simplicibus;* William of Saliceto, *Summa conservationis et curationis*, bk 4; Isaac, *Dietae particulares*, bk 1.

44   Henry of Huntingdon, *Anglicanus Ortus: A Verse Herbal of the Twelfth Century*, ed. and trans. Winston Black. Studies and Texts 180. British Writers of the Medieval and Early Modern Period 3. (Toronto: Pontifical Institute of Mediaeval Studies; Oxford, Bodleian Library, 2012).

45   *Alphita*, ed. Alejandro García González (Florence: SISMEL/Edizioni del Galluzzo, 2008).

46   Dietlinde Goltz, ed. *Mittelalterliche Pharmazie und Medizin: dargestellt an Geschichte und Inhalt des Antidotarium Nicolai* (Stuttgart: Wissenschaftliche Verlagsgesellschaft, 1976).

47   Maaike Van der Lugt, "'Abominable Mixtures': The 'Liber vaccae' in the Medieval West, or the Dangers and Attractions of Natural Magic," *Traditio* 64 (2009): 229–77.

48   See the remarks on "designer herbals" in Keiser, "Vernacular Herbals: A Growth Industry in Late Medieval England," in *Design and Distribution of Late Medieval Manuscripts in England*, ed. Margaret Connolly and Linne R. Mooney (Woodbridge: York Medieval Press, 2008), 304–6.

# PART TWO

# Texts and Legacy

*Chapter Four*

## Textual Layers in the *Liber Uricrisiarum*

E. RUTH HARVEY

The *Liber Uricrisiarum* was a highly conscious innovation in English writing. Henry Daniel was keenly aware that no one had ever done such a thing before and began by highlighting his own difficulties. The book was to comprehend a very large amount of Latin learning. It would require the crafting of a new vocabulary, and necessitate the introduction of a whole framework of scientific enquiry. It would introduce into English the learned treatise, with its divisions, arguments, cross-references, technical vocabulary, and annotations (inserted parenthetically in the text). Daniel also introduced something else: he subjected his work to a process of scholarly revision, so that under his hands it grew ever larger and more complicated as he struggled to explain things more clearly and introduce still more new sources and authorities. When it seemed to him that the subject required further knowledge from a related area, he toyed with the idea of writing another book about that. In at least one case, he kept his promise.[1]

The *Liber Uricrisiarum*, as we have it today, exists in some form or other in thirty-seven manuscripts and two prints. About nineteen of these are major manuscripts, neither abbreviated nor fragmentary. But the text they contain is very complicated. Daniel revised his book at least three times, perhaps four, and his copyists quite often did not stick to the same version throughout their task. What we have now are manuscripts representing not just various "editions" of the text, but manuscripts representing selected parts of different "editions" in one volume.

We have made a start at sorting out some of Daniel's methods of working. Since the *Liber Uricrisiarum* is very long and there are many copies, it is an enormous task, so what follows is still rather tentative. And I am ignoring for the purpose of this discussion the looming problem of Daniel's corresponding Latin treatise on uroscopy. We have a mid-fifteenth-century manuscript of this Latin text, properly attributed to Daniel,[2] and containing much the same material, in shorter form, as the *Liber Uricrisiarum*. The authorship would seem to be confirmed by Daniel's reference, in the Prologue to the English book, to his own Latin treatise on urines.[3] The difficulty lies in the fact that the Latin book contains materials from all versions of the English text, not just the earliest version. This means that either Daniel revised his Latin book alongside his English one, or that he deliberately omitted some of the material in the Latin from the earliest versions of his English book. The latter suggestion seems very unlikely: see the discussion below. The problem is too complex to deal with at this point.

The various layers within the English *Liber Uricrisiarum* may be sorted out by the helpful dates Daniel inserted into his text. The Prologue is particularly useful: there he has a phrase where he says how many years he has worked on his book, and this gets revised upwards in later versions. In the body of the text, in his long astronomical excursus, he actually notes the very year in which he is working. In the process of explaining how to determine a leap year he says, "we ben now in 1000 300 and 77 ʒere of Oure Lorde," and goes on to show how you must then divide the last number by four: if it won't divide evenly by four, it is not a leap year. In the Prologue in the manuscripts that have 1377 as the year of writing, Daniel says that he has been working on compiling his book for two years.

In other manuscripts the leap year passage has the date changed to 1378, and the note in the Prologue on the preparation time needed for the book reads three years. The whole Prologue has been revised after this, with some passages added and the paragraphs rearranged. One manuscript changes the number of years in the Prologue to five. Several others have a complete revision of the whole astronomy passage, where the precise reference to a date has been removed, but a lot more information has been added.

In addition, in the set of Latin verses that conclude the book (not included in all manuscripts) the date 1379 is given as the year when it was completed. A couple of subsequent lines, referring to the "great insurrection" (1381) and the earthquake (1382) are added in five manuscripts.

Matching these clues to the whole group of manuscripts suggests up to five different versions:

1 Proto-alpha: dated 1377, with two years' work given in the Prologue. This has the first version of the Prologue, with the smallest number of projected chapters. This text is contained in only two manuscripts, and runs only to Book 2.6, where the scribes switch to a different copy-text, so there are no concluding verses to this version.

2  First revision (a tentative category). This text is contained in four manuscripts, and includes the whole text, from the Prologue to the final verses (going up to the year 1379). It has the same Prologue as proto-alpha, with the same "two years" reference, but in the passage on leap years the date is changed to 1378.

3  The alpha text. This contains the whole revised text, with the internal date of 1378. However, the Prologue has also been revised and rearranged, and the time spent working on the book has been changed to three years. The alpha text, like the first revision, contains the whole work, and has 1379 in the final verses. In the alpha text we have edited in *Liber Uricrisiarum: A Reading Edition*, the Prologue has been translated from Latin into English.

4  The beta text. Here Daniel subjected his whole book to a major revision, notably changing all the chaptering so that the original fourteen chapters of alpha's Book 2 have now been broken down into about eighty much smaller chapters. The whole text has been worked over in detail, and there are very many important enlargements. There are four complete manuscripts of this text; two include the Prologue and final verses, but only one of the prologues includes the reference to the period of time spent working on the book as "5 years" (the other leaves a space). The verses end with the 1379 date.

5  The beta star, or revised beta text. This last version of the *Liber Uricrisiarum* exists only in its latter part: both the scribes who wrote out proto-alpha change their copy-text just after the astronomy passage, and continue with a text which seems to have even more revisions and additions than the beta text. Similarly, four of the scribes who started to write out the alpha text switch midway to beta star, though at different points in the text. Beta star has a good deal in common with the beta text, but there are some very interesting and important additions. Beta star texts usually have the Latin verses, and include the two lines that bring the latest date mentioned down to 1382.

Daniel's revisions to his text provide a good deal more insight into his thinking, as well as demonstrating how his ideas and style developed. The subject is a huge one, and I can offer only a few preliminary reflections here.

*1. Proto-alpha*

The first English version of the *Liber Uricrisiarum* is made up of the first version of the Prologue, the earliest version of Book 1 and the first six chapters of Book 2. It is contained in two manuscripts: Bodley e Musaeo

116 (M6), and Cambridge, Gonville & Caius 180/213 (G3); neither manuscript is a copy of the other, but they both share common errors, so
they must go back to a common original.[4] Both M6 and G3 switch the
copy-text in the course of Book 2 to the latest version of the text, the
revised beta text (which we are calling beta star). Both manuscripts are
very close to each other, but oddly, do not make the switch at precisely
the same place. Both scribes seem to have been slightly confused: M6
has a short overlap between versions, but does not signal any break in
the sense, whereas the G3 scribe copied the proto-alpha text up to the
same point, then jumped back to an earlier passage in the beta star text,
which covers some of the same ground he has already covered. After
a page or so he seems to have realised he was repeating the material,
stopped, left a leaf blank, and then rejoined beta star at the same point
as M6 does.

   This first version of the book is a bit sparser in vocabulary and detail.
Daniel divided his subject on conventional lines: there was to be one
book describing the *condiciones*, the considerations a physician should
bear in mind when examining a urine specimen; Book 2 was to be made
up of the twenty colours of urine, and Book 3 the nineteen or twenty
different "contents" of urine (such things as foam, blood, and gravel).
In the Prologue Daniel said that Book 1 was to have fourteen chapters
(this could be a mistake for four, as in the alpha version, but the two
copies both seem confused). M6 gives chapter numbers in the running
heads going up to 16; G3 has odd numbers in the margins, but very
inconsistently noted. Then the Prologue said Book 2 was to have nine
chapters, and Book 3, nineteen, but this scheme does not correspond at
all to the notations in the text. The scribe frequently leaves out chapter
numbers altogether: in Book 2 he forgot to enter chapter 3, although he
left a space for it; chapter 4 is there, but chapters 5 and 6 are signalled in
the running head, not numbered in the text. The digression on the planets is labelled *tractatio planetarum* and *materia planetarum* as a subhead-
ing to "cap. 5" in the running head. When the scribe shifts his copy-text,
he starts numbering chapters from 40 onwards, corresponding to most
of the beta manuscripts.

   From the beginning Daniel favoured a numbering scheme that was
characteristically complicated. He nested one numeration system
within another (thus in the alpha version the twenty *condiciones* are
all subsections of chapter 4 of Book 1). In nearly all the manuscripts
the scribes found this confusing, and were often tempted to number
the condiciones as if they were chapters. Nevertheless, the essential
scaffolding of the book is laid down in the proto-alpha version, which
gets enlarged and expanded in all sorts of ways, but does not depart in

essence from the fundamental three-part framework: three books devoted to the three divisions: *condiciones*, colours, contents.

## 2. The First Revision

What I am calling "the first revision" is perhaps not clearly separable from the alpha text, the one presented in our edition. I have separated the stages here because, while Daniel certainly revised the whole proto-alpha text with numerous small changes, in alpha proper he provided a revised Prologue in which he alters the time he has been working on the book to three years. The manuscripts that contain the "old" Prologue – fundamentally the same one found in proto-alpha – keep it at two years. There are four in all: the two related manuscripts Sloane 1100 and Sloane 1721 (Sa, Sc), Trinity College Cambridge MS O.12.21 (T), and Gloucester Cathedral MS 19 (G). These comprise what I have been calling "the first revision" group. The revision itself is much the same throughout this group and the alpha group. The "first revision" group, SaScTG, however, not only have the first Prologue in common, but are all in a distinct textual subgroup, marked out by minor common differences. It is possible that when Daniel rewrote the Prologue he stopped at that, though it seems uncharacteristic; but it would take a great deal of work to explore every variant to see if the new Prologue warrants the new category I am suggesting here. I will consider the main revisions under the next category, the alpha text.

## 3. The Alpha Text

The alpha text proper is the one we have edited from Royal MS 17 D.i (R) and e Musaeo 187 (M7). In these two manuscripts the text is complete, running from a new version of the Prologue (translated into English) to the final verses (although R has lost a few pages, including its final page). Other witnesses to the first half or so of the alpha text are the Huntington MS 505 and Boston P 361 manuscripts (H and B) and the two Cambridge University Manuscripts, CUL Ff.2.6 and Gg.3.29 (Cf and Cg). However, these last four manuscripts are hybrids: they contain the alpha text for the first part of the book, and then change, like the proto-alpha ones, but at different points, to a much later copytext. It could be argued that the alpha group is made up of all the manuscripts here and in the first revision category above, as well as R and M7. They all change the date in the astronomical passage to 1378, and they all share the same broad pattern of revision. But the alterations to the Prologue and the fact that RM7 and the first part of HBCfCg are textually all closer to each other, and differ from SaScGT in the same places, suggest that a distinction between the two groups should be explored.

For the alpha text, Daniel rewords a good number of phrases, very often providing more doublets and synonyms. For example, G3 reads:

> Some tyme þey pyssen os hyt were vyle rotyn blode, attyr & quitter, and sum tyme os hyt were blody mater, & sum tyme as hyt were rasyng of a byle or of a sore. Al ys bycause of hurtyng of þe vesice. (G3, f. 9v)[5]

In alpha this becomes:

> Somtyme þai pyssen as it were wel corupte and roten atter and quytter, somtyme as it were blody mater, & somtyme as it were þe scuddes and þe rasynges of a bile or of a sore, and all is be cause of scabihede and blemesshing of þe vessy. (R 1.4.101–5)

Daniel adds references, translates bits of Latin more regularly, and makes Latin and English equivalents more consistent; he provides English versions of Latin terms such as *jejunum, miseraice, lactea porta* ("jejune," "meseraice," "mylke ȝate"). References become more precise: "Gilbertus *in his coment vpon Giles*" (R 1.4.802); "What is mortificacioun Y saide *in þe nexte chapitle biforne*" (R 2.2.16–17). He elaborates on subjects that interest him, like the enquiry into the terms "diuretic" and "styptic": "Þus taȝght me one of þe wisest droggers of al Engelonde" (R 1.4.762–3), and adds random moral thoughts: "*Et* man schal lengh his lif for to leue and serue his God" (R 1.4.676–7). He indulges in his growing enthusiasm for etymologies: "And þis artarie þus at þe hert is called *adortus*, 'adort.' *Adortus*, i. *ad cor ortus* (*anglice*: spryngond at þe hert)" (R 2.3.105).

*4. The Beta Text*

The beta text, contained in Ashmole 1404 (A), Gonville and Caius 376/596 (G6), and the related pair, Wellcome 225 (W) and Egerton 1624 (E), has undergone a much more major revision. Daniel re-chapters the whole work, presumably to make details more accessible: some of his chapters in alpha were very long indeed; broken up, individual sections can be found much more quickly. He also adds large amounts of new material. The astronomical section grows much larger. He adds two more detailed case histories to illuminate his discussion of disease (see below). In Book 1 he brings in the amusing tale of Master Giles of Stafford, who supposedly diagnosed the pregnancies of a woman and her cow simultaneously, without even looking at the sample of their mixed urine she had brought him.[6] He elaborates the *condiciones*, bringing in the malady of *ereos* or love, and filling in the ones he had passed over more cursorily in proto-alpha and alpha. He adds a passage on pulses and one on faeces, and elaborates *pthisica*, women's problems, diabetes, and dropsy with much more information. He introduces an entirely new passage on the four kinds of leprosy. And throughout he indulges more in his twin passions for etymology and synonyms.

"Turbacioun of humores" (R 2.3.13) becomes "turbacioun, i of rollyng and hurlyng & distemperyng of the humores" (A, f. 38v). A typical example of Daniel's favourite words is alpha's "coagulacioun, i. þorgh coldehed and cluddyng of blode" (R 2.5.66). This becomes in beta: "coagulacioun of blod, i of mikel cold and of cruddyng and cloddyng of the blod" (A, f. 74r). (In Sb, which may here show a yet further revision, it runs: "coagulacion of blood i of mekyl cold and of cruddyng and cloddyng and clumperyng of þe blood," Sb, f. 82v.) *Arteria, peripulmonia, matrix, pthisis, ethica, ictericia, herpesestiomenum* all receive expanded etymologies.

## 5. The Beta Star Text

Beta star is the name we have been using for the section of text used to complete the manuscripts of proto-alpha, M6 and G3, which is also the text that scribes graft into some of the alpha texts (HBCgCf). We do not have a beginning to this revision. Our manuscripts begin part way through Book 2 and have different starting points. It has many small revisions, and some interesting larger additions, notably a whole section on bones (chapter 2.41 in G3M6Sb). The revisions are uneven: they range from simple additions, such as the bones, to more elaborate re-writings, such as the section on pthisis. Beta star continues to display Daniel's tendency to add in synonyms and new English terms: "smale particules, smale chyppynges" (A, f. 147r) become "lytyl smale chyppyngys, partyculys, smale offals" (M6, f. 129v). "Cold clatteth and clammeth it togedur" (A, f. 152v) appears as "colde clacchyþ and clammyth & clingyth hyt togydyr" (G3, f. 135r). "Lumpysh and clumpysh, cruddysh and spottysh" (A, f. 157r) becomes "clumperysch and cloddysche, craggysche and spottysche" (M6, f. 136v). In this last revision there are new citations of the *Rogerina magna*, which Daniel had introduced in the beta revision, and from Theophilus and Gilbert, new etymologies (*optalmia, artetica passio*), and still more personal remarks.

Two manuscripts that are difficult to classify perhaps belong here. Sloane 1101 (Sb) is largely a beta text, but it has some, though not all, of the enlargements in beta star: it does have the bones, for instance, and various extra phrases. Sb includes the long, highly astrological passage at the end of the astronomical section, which is also included by the otherwise beta text A. The other anomalous text, St John's College B.16 (J), appears to be an abbreviated version of Sb. Both manuscripts need further study.

The whole extent of Daniel's revisions to his text is too large to deal with here, but in notable areas they are particularly conspicuous. Four topics to which he returns over and over again are astronomy/astrology; the problem of pthisis and "hectic fever"; his own involvement in medicine; and the subject of women and sex.

### Astronomy/astrology

There is a lengthy section in the middle of the *Liber Uricrisiarum* that is devoted to "what a wise leche owe forto know" about the influence of the stars on the earth. Since it was an article of medieval science that the whole cosmos had a powerful effect on the central earth, this makes good medical sense, although Daniel in fact does not mention planetary influence anywhere else in his theory: it is confined entirely to this one long passage in the middle of the book. Even if he did not integrate astrological theory into his practical medicine, Daniel remained fascinated by it. The planetary passage undergoes expansion at all stages of the development of his text.

In the first version, proto-alpha, it occupies about six pages. The term "planetic fever," a wandering or irregular fever, introduces the word "planet"; and Daniel seizes upon the occasion to explain exactly how many planets there are, and how they affect the world beneath. He goes through the seven planets, taking the opportunity to explain, under Luna, the moon, what the zodiac is, and how time is divided up into days, hours, and degrees. Under Sol, the sun, he gives an explanation of leap years, and how to calculate them. This is where he gives the useful information that the year he is writing in is 1377. He gives two different ways of finding the "Sunday Letter" to work out the ecclesiastical calendar, and explains why there are differing numbers of days in the months. The other planets get shorter shrift: he covers Mercury, Venus, Mars, Jupiter, and Saturn in a paragraph each. Next, he lists the planetary "houses" or signs of the zodiac that they are associated with, classifies the signs to match the four qualities, and lists the parts of the body governed by the zodiacal signs. Since "astronomers" advise that

In the proto-alpha version pthisis appears in 2.3, "Blo colour." Essentially the urine is greyish and uneven-looking, with tiny clumps of bubbles in it, which points to the "airy" organ, the lungs. Pthisis is effectively a decaying of the lungs, *ulceracio pulmonis*; it occurs mostly in the young, those aged between eighteen and twenty-five, and the victims mostly do not live beyond thirty-five. Those of a certain bodily physique, thin and narrow-chested, are most prone to it. Their spittle smells evil, some will die soon, and some will suffer for years, because, once present, the disease is incurable. If there is hair loss or dysentery, it will soon be fatal. Daniel mentions, but does not connect, the spitting of blood as a symptom at this point.

Hectic fever is a subset of pthisis: it is what used to be known as "galloping consumption," the rapidly progressing last stages of tuberculosis. Daniel says it arises as the result of a longstanding condition: overwork, or strain, too much studying, or bad dieting, or lechery. The body is now in such a degraded state that it cannot recover, and it will gradually be consumed by a low fever, which remorselessly burns its way through the tissues.[10] He concludes the passage by distinguishing three "kinds" or stages of hectic fever, marked by increasing heat, dryness, thirst, and last of all, by the complete loss of elasticity in the skin: "yf þu lyfte vp hys skynne it goþ not doun aȝen pleyn os it was but it be put doun aȝen wt an hond" (M6, f. 86r).

In the next version of the text, the first revision, there are the usual small expansions of phrases, translations, and cross references, but when Daniel reaches the passage on hectic fever he imports a paragraph of symptoms from later on in his book: hot hands and feet, flushed cheeks, cough, and a steady burning fever, which the patient cannot perceive. That the whole paragraph was included twice in the first revision texts – here and in chapter 10 on Rufus urine – suggests that these "hot" symptoms first struck Daniel as being characteristic of a hot fever, but he had begun to connect them with the much "colder" disease, pthisis. The alpha text proper completed the re-think by moving the passage entirely to Blo, and does not repeat it under Rufus.

In the beta revision, he changed his mind again, and moved the paragraph on symptoms back to Rufus. The rest of the text has been reworked and often reworded, and there are enlargements where Daniel worries about etymologies and disambiguation of terms ("Lateyn hath many vnstedfaste knokkeris at his gate," A, f. 51v; Sb, f. 56v). Then he adds an elaboration to his note on the deadly effect of a flux on those suffering from "rooted pthisis."

In the beta star revision, the subject of pthisis and hectic fever is, as in the beta version, covered under Rufus, but there are yet more additions. He adds to the list of symptoms, noting that the fingernails of consumptives are characteristically deformed; and includes an entirely new paragraph on the reason for the faint traces of fat in the urine of those with hectic fever. In turn, the chapter on fat in urine in Book 3 has been adjusted to cross-reference this paragraph.[11]

In the beta text Daniel had also revisited his chapter on Pallid urine to bring out much more firmly that ashy residue in the urine is again a symptom of pthisis; it is another indication that a slow fever is burning away the tissue of the lungs. He goes back to this again in beta star, and adds a note that the bones in the breast are particularly susceptible to heat, which lingers there and dries out the lungs. He cross-references this remark back to what he said in Blo colour.

This continual revision and reworking of the same subject are characteristic of Daniel at his best. He was determined to give the most complete and up-to-date theoretical account of medical problems. His handling of tuberculosis demonstrates his anxiety to get it right, to sort out the "hot" and "cold" aspects of the disease, and to put the information in its most useful place, complete with cross-references back and forth, to "fat," to the anatomical section in Karopos, to the various colours that might be relevant. It seems that he came by more information on, for instance, the significance of fatty residue in urine, and did some of the rewriting to incorporate it into his diagnosis and theory. He continually refined his statements, his organization, and his references to represent the best information he could find. Pthisis and hectic fever provide a good example of his engagement, research, and scholarship.

### Daniel's Own Medicine

One of the more significant developments in the *Liber Uricrisiarum* concerns Daniel's own personal experience of medicine and medical practice. In the earliest version of the book, apart from the Prologue, Daniel keeps himself mostly in the background. He acknowledges his sources conscientiously, quoting "worde for worde," citing and translating individual aphorisms and phrases in Latin. But as he revises, he allows himself more involvement. Most conspicuously in the beta revision he illustrates his points by introducing case histories of actual patients. "Also I knew by a wydowe, nerhand of 60 ȝer of age, & her husbond eke, and thei wer worthi folke" (A, f. 59r),[12] he says, apropos of a citation of Aristotle on a phantom pregnancy, and goes on to describe what she told him, and what her neighbours thought, about her own similar case. "I wiste where a woman was, a worthy wyfe skantely of 30 yere age" (A, f. 63v) in a case of dropsy, and records the various opinions of her physicians and bystanders, "me present." A third example, the case of the young man of Stamford, first appeared in the first revision text. It is recorded impersonally, but the circumstantial details suggest that Daniel had witnessed it himself.[13] (Since Daniel regarded himself primarily as an herbalist, one might speculate that he was the one who recommended the use of "pety bugle" to the patient, who dosed himself with it "os he was taght" (A, f. 97v–98r).) It is curious that this last anecdote, the first 'case history' to be included in the *Liber Uricrisiarum*, was deliberately omitted from the last version. Both proto-alpha texts, which at this point have switched their copy-manuscripts to a beta star witness, include only a notation, *"de narracione,"* to mark the omission, and patch up the sentence at the end to make the new transition work. All three anecdotes first appear together in the beta text, and are carefully linked to the subject: the phantom pregnancy bears out Aristotle; the dropsical woman is introduced to illustrate an outstanding example of the disease; and the noteworthy colour of the urine of the man from Stamford illustrates very clearly a point Daniel was making about the relative "thickness" of *karopos* urine.

Galen frequently included case histories in his works, so there was good medical precedent; but it does bring the author more into the foreground as a self-proclaimed authority. Daniel's inclusion of such anecdotes appears along with the introduction of a number of personal comments in the beta text, which could also be seen as a sign of his growing self-confidence. He notes at one point that he would like to give more information, but he lacks the most up-to-date books, Bernard of Gordon's *Lilium medicine* and Lanfranc's work, "ne such oder new auctores for fawte of pecuny may not getyn ʒow; þowh I wold; yitt I wote well where thei be & pore & simple hath litel wok <='power'>" (A, f. 45r). He seems to have got hold of the text called *Rogerina magna* by the time he made the beta revision; there he uses it to import a lengthy passage on the four kinds of leprosy, and adds it as an authority in a note in beta star 3.3 (Cg, f. 129r).

In another case of updating his material, somewhere between the alpha text and the beta revision he revised his classification of the kinds of dropsy (alpha 2.3; beta 2.16). At first he had said there were three kinds, *leucofleuma, alchites,* and *tympanides.* In beta he adds a lengthy passage beginning, "Sum seyn thus, and better to me, that there be 4 spices of ydropisy and thus is her speche" (A, f. 62r). The four kinds of dropsy now include *yposarcha,* and match the four humours more neatly.

In the first version of the Prologue Daniel adopted a humble and dutiful pose: he is just trying to serve his fellow man. In the alpha revision, however, he has become rather less *faux*-humble, promising worldly success, among other things, to his faithful readers. He also adds the promise that, God willing, he will write another book about medicines to cure the maladies the *Liber Uricrisiarum* diagnoses. This presages a series of remarks in which Daniel reveals his ambitions, and perhaps his achievements, in the authorial role. One is to write the astronomy text mentioned above (in a beta star witness). In the course of the beta revision he also alludes to his ambitions to write a book on pulses and other bodily signs (A, f. 36v), and feels that one on the crisis is needed (A, f. 34r). In the beta star revision of 3.1, he directs his readers to consult his own *practica* on medicine: "*Cassia fistula, se in our practyke*" (G3, f. 123r).

More entertainingly, Daniel appears more and more in his own book in the form of personal comments, small insults, and snide remarks. For instance, when he gets to kidney disease in beta star (3.5) he adds the comment, "nefresy, gret and huge dissese, and þys fele I well also in my self alle tymys of þe ȝere continuelly" (M6, f. 129v). This seems to be a growing tendency: he sometimes makes similar personal comments in his herbal, which he wrote after the *Liber Uricrisiarum*. As for disparaging remarks, in proto-alpha 2.4 (G3, f. 50r–v) he writes, "myche folke and many vnwyse lechys wenun and demun þat [colic] for þe ston." The alpha text converts the unwise into the professionally inept: "mykel folk & also many entermetours of lechecrafte wene & deme it for þe ston" (R 2.4.178–9). In the beta text they have turned into "bunglers and smatterers": "mikel folke and many vnwyse leches as thes bugeres <*miswritten for* bunglers? jangelers W> & smatterers" (A, f. 68r). In beta star they are "many onwyse lechys – as þese boungleres and smatereres of þe craft [who] – wenyn and demyn it for *calculus*" (Sb, f. 76r). Daniel clearly enjoyed elaborating his phrases.

Daniel must have met more annoying practitioners later on. In the alpha text of 3.19 there are two innocuous sentences:

And som saie þat wan whit colour in ypostasi or in vryn, wheþer it be, it seiþ bigynnyng of digestioun. Anoþer maner of whitehede þere is in ypostasy and in vryn: þat is brigh mylk white. (R 3.19.46–9)

But in the beta revision a new sentence is inserted beween them:

But ofte tymes whitehed in vryn or in ypostasy is taken for yolowyshed and for very whitehed among thes dog leches, and among them þat haue not perfyte vnderstondyng, that hath sen litel and speken mikel, and wold be sen and mow not for pride and dulhed lerne, as many of my order. (A, f. 173v and all beta versions)

In beta star the dog leeches are also ignorant smatterers, but the gibe against friars has gone:

> But take hede þat oftuntyme whytysched in vryn or in ipostasi is takyn for ȝelowysched and sumty <sic> for very whithed amonge dogge lechys and smaterers and hem þat ben suche lechis þat lytil han seyn and lytill kunne. (M6, f. 145v)

Either Daniel thought better of it, or perhaps a scribe removed it. The fact that two of the beta star witnesses (HG3) added "etc" after "kunne" rather suggests it was a scribe who removed the insult.

## Women and Sex

One last major area where Daniel continually adjusted his text is, rather surprisingly for a friar, his treatment of women and sexual topics. Women's issues come up several times: the major passages are in Book 2.3, Blo colour, where he discusses the uterus and its maladies; and in Book 3.16, on *attomi* or Motes, where he explains the signs of pregnancy evidenced by motes in the urine. There is a very brief list of the sexual organs, male and female, under Book 2.7, Karopos, with the addition of some rude English verses (based distantly on Prov 30 15–16) on the insatiability of the *os vulvae*. The scribes of two manuscripts (A and M6) leave the verses out.

The passage dealing with ailments of the *matrix* or womb (2.3) undergoes revisions at all stages. At first, Daniel explains what the womb is: he thinks it is woolly inside, and has seven compartments; from the outside it looks like a grain of wheat. The first and most significant malady discussed is menstruation: a phenomenon caused by the fundamental female qualities of coldness and moistness. A woman's coldness means she cannot rid her body of impurities; hence these gather in the womb and are emitted once a month. Daniel points out that menstrual blood is poisonous to men, trees, and dogs.

Then he describes the act of copulation, and tells how the matrix seals itself up once it has received the semen. Conception makes a woman much warmer, so her menses dry up, and instead serve to nourish the foetus. A woman has "testicles" too, but they are inside her body, and the foetus is made up of both kinds of sperm, which ought to be emitted simultaneously in coitus. The sex of the infant is determined by where in the womb it develops: if it lodges in a right-hand compartment it develops in a warmer environment, and therefore turns into a boy. Colder girls develop on the colder side of the body. The middle compartments produce more ambiguous children, such as "faint-hearted" boys and "bold and sturdy" girls. The foetus grows inside a membrane that Daniel calls the secundine, which emerges with the baby. He cites a very popular dictum from St Augustine on the various stages of development of the foetus, and adds Aristotle's view that males acquire "life and movement" in forty days; females in eighty.

Daniel is troubled throughout the whole passage by his belief that women are most lecherous when they are most poisonous, i.e., when they are menstruating, and that they do not cease to desire sex when they are pregnant, unlike the other animals. He tries to explain this, but it is clearly bothersome. He returns to the topic in his discussion of conception in 3.16.

The specific problems with the uterus are first given, in proto-alpha, as its tendency to wander around inside the woman. Again, the problem is chiefly cold: the uterus moves around seeking warmth. If it gets really cold it suffers from *syncopis*, which causes the woman to collapse, curl up, grind her teeth, lose speech, and die. This terrible disease often afflicts those without a man, widows, young unmarried girls, and wives with absent husbands: they desperately need to rid themselves of their own cold sperm, or to acquire some hot male sperm to counteract their dangerous coldness. Daniel concluded the passage with a note on the age at which menopause might be expected, and notes that postmenopausal women are more likely to suffer from movements of the uterus. He adds a remark about women's extreme secretiveness about these matters: they "raþer dyen þeron þan tellyn hyt any man for shame."

In the alpha version Daniel touches up this material with many small details, phrases, and clarifications, and refers his readers to Aristotle's *History of Animals* for more information, "which I passe because of prolixite." But in the major beta revision he goes over it all again, with larger additions. There are etymologies, and more comments; more illnesses, such as retention of the menses, or excessive or painful menses. Aristotle's account of a *mola matricis*, a monstrous lump in the womb that resembles pregnancy, is recorded in detail. Daniel then supplies his own story of his acquaintance, the old widow who claimed to have been pregnant for twenty-three years. He adds an extra passage on the pains of childbirth, and some of its difficulties. He points out that good care should be taken of pregnant women, and that an expert midwife is a necessity.

We do not have a beta star text for this passage – it is too early in the text, but the anomalous manuscript, Sloane 1101 (Sb), which might here reflect a lost beta star text, gives yet another, longer, reworking of

Aristotle's passage on *mola matricis,* to stress that it proves that women need special care right from the time they conceive. Sb, incidentally, provides another vernacular name for *mola matricis*: "þat þei callyn þe elvysch kechil or þe elvysch cake" (Sb, f. 67r).[14]

Daniel's interest in lechery and its effects is abiding throughout the *Liber Uricrisiarum.* Lechery gets cited more and more often as the precipitating cause of various maladies, notably diabetes, where he is moved in the beta revision to add a helpful list of the number of times men should indulge in sexual activity according to their age; by the time they reach sixty, for example, they should have sex only once or twice over a period of three months. But his moral desire to disparage lust is in interesting contrast with his medical belief that sexual activity is necessary to health. He is clear from the beginning that, whatever its moral status, the organs of males and females need each other. The clearest statement of this occurs in one of the proto-alpha texts in 1.4 *condicio 7*:

> For euery man is kyndely hott & drye of kynde, and euery womman cold & moyst of kynde. And þat is þe cause why womman desyryth so man & why man desyry3th so womman, for euery qualyte wolde be refresschyd with oþyr. (M6, f. 71r)

The naturally cold *matrix* is made for the naturally hot *yerd*; and the obviousness of this is reinforced with an etymology provided in the last, beta star text:

> *vulua* ys the wombe gate and the gate of oure kynde, dicitur a *volo, -is*; for all men, be they neuer so good in lyuynge, if they were sykyr to skapyn harmylese both of God and of man and of all the world, they wulde hyt and desyre hyt kyndely. Also of *volo, vis,* 'to wylle,' for the membre and the beste that beryth hyt wolde all more, for wery they mown been, bot anowh mow they not haue. (G3, 2.7 f. 80v–81r)

The underlying conflict between the pious disapproval of sexual activity and the medical realities of erotic desire reaches its unexpected resolution in the development of a particular statement towards the end of the book.

Daniel embarked on the subject of pregnancy with a citation of St Paul, "to the pure all things are pure" to justify his detailed disquisitions.[15] Most scribes copied them without demur. But his most striking passage was completely elided by the most squeamish scribe, the one who copied M6, though it occurs in the closely related manuscripts, G3 and BHCg. In alpha 3.16, where Daniel is recording the signs of pregnancy, the first sign of all must be learned by asking the woman to lay bare the intimate moments of her most recent sexual encounter "with man þat is myghty for to gendren" (R 3.16.234–5). Her answer will enable the physician to determine if she has conceived. In alpha the physician must enquire:

> If sche conceyued when she was laste servede, her matrice drowe & soke his ȝerde, os a water leche sokeþ on a man, or best on þe moder pappe, in so mykel þat þe man þoght þat þe womannes membre soke and drowe his ȝerde awaie fro him. (R 3.16.243–6)

This stays much the same throughout all the earlier versions – except that the Royal scribe leaves out a concluding phrase, "and namely if his yerd be long," which appears in all the other versions after proto-alpha, except for RM7. The beta revision alters this to "and namely if his yerd be grete or long or els bothe" (A, f. 166v). But beta star reworks the whole passage in detail:

> If she conceyvyd whan she was laste served of man her matrice wythin her bodye haled and drowe and soked the mans yerde ende, right as a chyld or a beste on þe moder pappe, or as a water leche on a mans legge to sowke the blood, or as a lampray on a stone to sowke his food, in so mo-che that the man thynkyth to his felynge or perceyvyng, for the whyle and the tyme, that she sowkyth and drawith his yerde, and namely his yerde ende, away fro hym, and namely yf hys yerde be so longe or so grete or bothe. And yet his lykynge lasteth all that whyle that she soketh so. (Cg, f. 156r–156v)

Here Daniel is developing the ideas expressed earlier in his book about the naturalness of desire, and the nature of the matrix in 2.3. His conviction that conception required a certain enthusiasm on the part of the matrix gets stronger in each revision. In the beta version he claimed that the matrix holds on to the "yerd end" so strongly that it is hard to separate a couple locked in coital union: "it shuld be a strong pulle and a myghty that shuld hem atwynne" (A, f. 55r).

From the first, in proto-alpha, he had insisted that the male and female sperms should be harmonious in temperament for conception to take place. In the beta revision he elaborates this to claim that the seed must be not only of the correct temperament, but both parties should reach sexual climax almost at once, so that the sperms can unite in generation: "for hem muste yeve bothe at oons or els he firste & she sone after, while the matrice soketh as I seide" (A, f. 55v). In the beta star revision, Daniel reiterates the same ideas, even repeating some of the same words, in his *Attomi* chapter in Book 3.

There is another development. The second thing the physician must ask the woman is about the present state of her own sexual organs; because, if she is pregnant,

> her wombe ȝate boketh noght ne bolketh ne openeth þe self, ne is noȝt so wete ne so wosie, ne giffeth noght so mykel of moystur oute, i.e. soueriþ noȝt ne is noght so woode to lecherie os it was biforn. & þat is bi cause þat þe seede of man is receyuede in þe matrice and þe matrice is fedde & fild þerwiþ and her þirst of lecherie is quenchede þat biforne myght noght cessen. For meny wemen ar neuer ful til þai have conceyuede, and þerfor sche is noght so woode in hereselfe to swich dede as sche was biforn. (R 3.16.246–53)

The beta text rewords this again, adding the phrase, "but it is drye and wel" in the middle, after "biforn." And in beta star he adds a final touch, at the end:

> And also therwyth his yerde ende be drye as he had nought don so, for his ful kynde for the tyme is spurged in her. And so eyther hath made a sethe to other, and bothe arn in pees. (Cg, f. 156v)

To "make a sethe," or "make asseth" is a fairly rare term from the fourteenth century, meaning "to give satisfaction."[16] Here Daniel's endorsement of sexual pleasure, mutuality, and contentment, prevails over his worries about "lechery." And it is interesting that he continued, throughout his revisions, in making the emphasis stronger.

It was too much for one of his scribes. M6 omits the whole passage and starts with the second sign of conception, cessation of the menses, although the closely related text in G3 has the whole piece. M6 had been similarly squeamish about the description of the sexual organs in beta star, Book 2 (M6, 2.44 f. 105v, under Karopos): he simply goes as far as the reference back to Blo colour, and omits everything, including the antifeminist verses, to the end of the chapter (A also omitted the verses, but retained the anatomy). Perhaps if he were copying the text for a monastery, a scribe might feel some things were unnecessary and unseemly; but Daniel, himself a friar, clearly had more on his mind than a clerical audience.

## Conclusion

Reading Daniel's *Liber Uricrisiarum* in all its different versions is a fascinating exercise. It lets us in to some of his thought processes, to his development as a scholar and a writer, to his increasing range and ambition. Far too long dismissed as a mere translation of Isaac Judaeus, the *Liber Uricrisiarum* is a monumental work of its time: completely unparalleled in English in the fourteenth century. Daniel's engagement with his project never ceased. He carried on reading more, updating, adjusting, and elaborating. There was perhaps no last word: the *Liber Uricrisiarum* remained a work in progress right until the end.

NOTES

1 His herbal, analysed by Winston Black in this volume, "Translation, Comparison, and Adaptation: Latin Verse Herbals in the *Aaron Danielis*," 38–62. This is what the "book of remedies" promised in the Prologue (*unum opus ad hoc me facturum promitto*) seems to be. Perhaps the same work mentioned in Sb, f. 8v: "of þese soris & siknesse, & of alle þat arn towchid in þese 3 bookes & in alle þe siknessis in mannys body þat I may fyndyn in phisik see in owre praptyk." For another projected work, see Sb, f. 41v: "For to spekyn of powses, it askith a book be þe self, and al a doyng be þe self. For on craft of leche craft þat is be demyng of sey3te in a mannys face, a noþer doyng be spatle of mowth, a noþer be powsis, and þe ferthe be þe egestioun of man, and alle I wolde undon in comoun speche, þat alle men my3tyn understonden and knowe, if ony man wolde fynde me myn sustenance."
2 Glasgow, Glasgow University Library, MS Hunter 362.
3 "I haue gadrede now late for þam þat kan take it in Latyn a schorte tretice conteynyng fully þe marowe of þis faculte" (Pro.79–81).
4 There also is a small fragment of Daniel's text with the same 1377 date in the leap-year discussion in Sloane 134, ff. 9r–20v. M. Teresa Tavormina also discusses Sloane 134 and its sibling, Sloane 2527, in her chapter in this volume.
5 This passage also appears in M6, f. 69v.
6 For a discussion of this tale, see Hannah Bower's chapter in this volume, "'Her ovn self seid me': The Function of Anecdote in Henry Daniel's *Liber Uricrisiarum*," 133–57.
7 See the astrological texts discussed in *Popular and Practical Science of Medieval England*, ed. Lister M. Matheson (East Lansing, Colleagues Press, 1994), and those printed in *Sex, Aging & Death in a Medieval Medical Compendium:*

*Trinity College Cambridge MS R.15.42, Its Texts, Language, and Scribe,* ed. M. Teresa Tavormina, 2 vols. (Arizona Center for Medieval and Renaissance Studies, 2006).

8   See Tavormina's discussion of this manuscript in "The Heirs of Henry Daniel: The Fifteenth- and Sixteenth-Century Legacy of the *Liber Uricrisiarum,*" 108–32 of this volume.

9   Daniel's material has a lot in common with the texts printed in Lynn Thorndike, *The Sphere of Sacrobosco and its Commentators* (Corpus of mediaeval scientific texts, Mediaeval Academy of America and the University of Chicago, v. 2.), 1949. See also the detailed commentary to *Liber Uricrisiarum* 2.6, ff. 146.

10   There is another beta star addition on the "lent fever" of consumption in 2.40 (M6, f. 110r): noting that its main effect is to dry out the lungs.

11   Daniel seems to have become interested in the whole question of fat or oil in urine and its connection to tuberculosis, somewhere in between beta and the beta star revision. He adjusts his chapter on Nubes in urine in Book 3 to suggest that it can be a form of *urina oleagina* (M6 131r), and is "þe fyrste and þe prynspal tokun toward þe etyke"; there are also a number of revisions in the whole chapter on *pinguedo.*

12   Quoted from A, f. 59r with "80 ȝer" emended to "60 ȝer" (SbW).

13   All of these examples are analysed fully in their narrative context in Hannah Bower's chapter in this volume. See Bower, "The Function of Anecdote," 133–57.

14   The only other examples of the term "elf-cake" in *OED* are recorded from 16th c., and there refer to a palpable enlargement of the spleen; s.v. Elf 6. For more on the "elvysch cake," see Sarah Star, "*Anima Carnis in Sanguine Est*: Life, Blood, and *The King of Tars,*" *Journal of English and Germanic Philology* 115.4 (2016): 442–62.

15   See *Epistle of Paul to Titus* 1:15. It is added, for example, to the text in G3, f. 81r, a beta star text by this point.

16   *MED s.v.* "asseth," n. 1.a).

*Chapter Five*

# The Heirs of Henry Daniel: The Fifteenth- and Sixteenth-Century Legacy of the *Liber Uricrisiarum*

M. TERESA TAVORMINA

## Introduction

One of the most familiar methods of measuring the contemporary success of a medieval work is by the number of surviving copies of the text. Even allowing for differential survival rates for different types of text, we usually take the survival of dozens of copies as a sign that a work was well-regarded by at least several generations of readers. Another touchstone by which we can judge contemporary esteem for a given work or author is imitation and extrapolation from the work in question – signs that the original continued to have influence both on its own and in its progeny.

Measured by its nineteen to twenty surviving complete or likely originally complete copies,[1] Henry Daniel's massive *Liber Uricrisiarum* (composed and revised ca. 1377–82) certainly qualifies as a successful piece of medical prose in its own right. When one adds the score of manuscripts that preserve excerpts, condensations, and adaptations of the text, Daniel's treatise rises into the top five most frequently copied and/or reworked Middle English uroscopies.[2]

This chapter surveys these reworkings of Daniel's text, the fifteenth- and sixteenth-century "heirs" of his trail-blazing introduction of medical concepts, information, and terminology in English at a time when the late-fourteenth-century burgeoning of Middle English scientific and medical prose had only barely begun.[3] After starting with Daniel's own modifications of and references to his text, the chapter proceeds from short extracts of the *Liber Uricrisiarum* and supplements to the full work, on to longer extracts from individual books, and finally to adaptations of the complete text. It thereby complements Peter Jones's chapter (63–83 above) on contemporary and later members of "this extraordinary generation" of English medical writers in both Latin and the vernacular.

## I. Daniel as His Own First Heir

*The Beta Version of the* Liber Uricrisiarum

The first significant adaptation of the *Liber Uricrisiarum* was Daniel's own revision, in what members of the Henry Daniel Project call the "beta version" of the *Liber Uricrisiarum*. As Harvey shows in chapter 4 above, Daniel was an inveterate reviser of his own work, and one family of witnesses is marked by several substantial additions[4] and a major change in the chaptering system, as well as numerous smaller additions, omissions, and revisions of shorter passages and phrasing. The re-chaptering involves converting the often very long chapters of the alpha version to many shorter chapters in the beta version. This restructuring is of particular interest because it may have been intended to make finding cross-referenced materials easier, by limiting the amount of text one would need to search to find a particular passage.

Unfortunately, scribes seem to have had a great deal of difficulty in copying the new chapter numbers accurately or completely, and several beta witnesses simply give up numbering chapters entirely or do so in a hit-or-miss fashion that makes the cross-references even more difficult to track down. As we will see, some of Daniel's later adapters appear to have abandoned the short-chapter system even though they are clearly working from a beta original.

*The Latin Version of the* Liber Uricrisiarum

In addition to the English versions of the *Liber Uricrisiarum*, Daniel wrote a condensed version in Latin, which survives in a single manuscript, Glasgow, University Library, MS Hunter 362 (L).[5] This redaction has the feel of a personal copy, almost a "file copy," containing the most important information from the more expansive English text. It should probably be identified with the "tractatum brevem (totam) huius facultatis medullam (plenius) continentem" written "in lingua vtique mihi cara" mentioned in all three versions of Daniel's Latin Prologue (= "a schorte tretice conteynyng fully þe marowe of þis faculte" in the English Prologue). The text includes a number of beta additions, including the story of Master Giles of Stafford (Book 1), lovesickness (*hereos*) under the condition Cura (Book 1),[6] the seven climates in the astro-calendric digression in Book 2, and the leprosy material under the colour Rubeus. Despite a brief Prologue that promises a beta-like chapter-structure (nineteen chapters in Book 1, ten [*lege* 80?] in Book 2, and thirty-three in Book 3), however, the actual chaptering is closer to that of the alpha text (2:11:18).

*Citations of the* Liber Uricrisiarum

One might have expected a text that was copied as often as the *Liber Uricrisiarum*, frequently with the author's name in its explicit, to be cited by other English medical writers, but such writers were probably more likely to invoke Latin authorities than their fellow vernacularisers.[7] The only direct medieval references to the *Liber Uricrisiarum* identified to date are those made in Daniel's own later works. Daniel's herbal treatise, which survives in only two mid-fifteenth-century manuscripts (London, British Library, Additional MS 27329 and the incomplete Arundel MS 42), frequently refers its readers to "oure *Uricrisis*" or simply "*Uricrisis*," with sufficient book and chapter detail to allow identification of the work with the revised, beta version of the *LU*. An incomplete astrological text in London, Wellcome Library MS 411 (s. xv[4/4]), ff. 9v–18v, the *Book of Nativities*, refers twice to a work called *Liber Vricrosiarum* and *Boke of Vricrosiarum* (f. 10v); the second of the references occurs with first-person attribution: "And begyn to rekene [the planetary hours] at mydneyght for þe skelys ["skills, reasons"] þat I seyde in þe boke of vricrosiarum."[8]

## II. Short Excerpts from the *Liber Uricrisiarum*

In two manuscripts, both medical miscellanies (London, British Library, Sloane MS 5 [s. xv[med]]; Cambridge, Magdalene College, MS Pepys 1661 [s. xv[1/2]]), we find passages on the planets taken from the astronomical and calendric digression in the alpha version of Daniel's treatise (R, 2.6.130–496).

*London, British Library, Sloane MS 5*

Sloane 5 (Sh) extracts paragraphs on the seven planets, focusing on their primary qualities, good or evil nature, appearance in the sky, influence on human beings, orbital periods, and length of time in each zodiacal sign (ff. 179v–181r). It omits material from the same passage on the natural day and its temporal divisions, astronomical units, and the calculation of leap year and dominical letters. The adapter of this passage clearly wanted a text focused on planets alone, which was then incorporated into a longer series of astronomical and medical texts within Sloane 5 (ff. 173r–190r), including lunary texts; the Daniel extract; several chapters on planets, elements, humours, complexions, and uroscopy drawn from an astromedical compendium found in Sloane 213 and other manuscripts;[9] and finally half a dozen additional Middle English uroscopies.

*Cambridge, Magdalene College, MS Pepys 1661*

The compiler of Pepys 1661 (Pe) gives the lion's share of that manuscript to recipe collections, along with a Middle English surgical treatise and various herbal texts at the end of the volume. The Vade Mecum Suite of brief uroscopy texts (*Twenty Colours by Digestion Groups, Urina Rufa,* and *Cleansing of Blood*) is embedded in one of the receptaria (the *Treasure of Poor Men,* pp. 22–8). The excerpt from Daniel (pp. 235–40) appears just before the sequence of herbal texts and is the only astronomical treatise in the manuscript; it is unusual within its manuscript for its non-therapeutic focus, although there is a brief text on perilous days, in a different hand, a few pages before it. There is no significant condensation of the original in the excerpt, but the copyist introduces or retains an unusual number of notable errors, especially in dates and other numerical details.

The Pepys extractor/compiler begins with the Sun and includes the leap year discussion, but specifies the current date as 1392 instead of the 1377 or 1378 found in Daniel's alpha version witnesses.[10] The extract ends just after Saturn, with the promise of a "rounde sercle" that will show the planetary and elemental spheres, the zodiacal signs, and the signs in which each planet reigns. Though no diagram follows, the intended "sercle" must have been the *rota celi* figure found or planned at this point in many copies of the *LU*; the lower portion of the page, about eleven lines long, has been left blank and could have held a smallish wheel of heaven.

**III. Supplements to the *Liber Uricrisiarum***

Whereas Sloane 5 and Pepys 1661 insert short passages from the *Liber Uricrisiarum* into medical miscellanies, the story changes when we turn to London, British Library, Sloane MS 1721 (ca. 1475) and Egerton MS 1624 (s. xv^med). Each of these manuscripts contains a complete or nearly complete copy of the *Liber Uricrisiarum* itself, with a few pages of supplemental uroscopic and other medical material added after the text; in Egerton 1624, several Latin and English texts are also inserted at the beginning and in the middle of the *LU*.

*London, British Library, Sloane MS 1721*

In Sloane 1721 (Sc), a witness to the alpha version, the added text is written in a sixteenth-century hand on a gathering of four smaller leaves at the end of the volume (ff. 214–17, the last leaf blank). The addendum describes the colours of urine in general and black urine in particular, with titles for the two topics that echo the chapter titles of *Liber Uricrisiarum* Book 2, chapters 1 and 2. The writer abridges and modernises the language of Daniel's original,[11] breaking off just before the section of chapter 2 on critical days. The abridgement process reduces the source passages substantially: Book 2.1 is shortened to about 29 per cent of its original length, while the first 2,360 words of Book 2.2 are reduced to some 1,060 words, or roughly 45 per cent of the original length.[12]

One minor peculiarity of the addendum occurs on the last three lines of f. 216r and all of 216v, where the scribe uses an easily decoded cipher for grammatical function words and the more substantive terms *vryn* and *blak*. None of the ciphered words and phrases is taboo, so the purpose of the ciphering remains unclear.

*London, British Library, Egerton MS 1624*

The compiler(s) of Egerton 1624 (E) created a fascinating framework for a beta copy of the *Liber Uricrisiarum* that is its primary text, a framework worth more extensive study than can be provided here. The *Liber Uricrisiarum* copy in Egerton 1624 was written by at least four different scribes,[13] with a near-contemporary foliation on most of the leaves containing Daniel's text. Other scribes may have written some or all of the non-Daniel passages.

A table of contents for the *Liber Uricrisiarum* begins on ff. 12v–13v and continues on ff. 213v–214r; it is cross-referenced to the old folio numbers and appears to be in the same hand as those numbers. Other additions include an English lyric on false friends; a Latin-French-English synonymy, mainly herbal; Latin texts on visiting the sick, treating them, and prognosticating life or death; three astro-calendric insertions in the middle and at the end of the manuscript, the first in Latin and the other two in English; miscellaneous recipes in later hands (Latin and English); and several short medical items at the end of the manuscript, including a unique English versification of John of Burgundy's four-chapter plague treatise, illustrated with a male figure depicting locations for purging plague buboes by bleeding,[14] as well as a hitherto-unidentified English translation of Bernard de Gordon's chapter on contents in urine (for verbal parallels supporting this identification, see Appendix 1, p. 125 below).

The astro-calendric insertions reveal careful reading of the *Liber Uricrisiarum* and what appears to be recognition of one of Daniel's key sources. The first insert is a parchment booklet (ff. 109–21; the only vellum in the manuscript), written entirely in Latin and with contents typical of both Latin and vernacular medical "almanacs," including eclipse tables for 1433–73. The booklet is inserted directly after the *rota celi* diagram (f. 108v) that concludes Daniel's discussion of astronomy and the calendar; it is not included in the old folio sequence, perhaps indicating a mid-fifteenth-century joining of the paper and parchment portions of the manuscript.

A second calendar-related insert appears on ff. 126–7, following a textual break that Egerton 1624 shares with London, Wellcome Library, MS 225 (W; ca. 1425), a close relative in the beta tradition. In the Wellcome manuscript, this textual break is followed by two originally blank pages (ff. 69–70), but in Egerton it is followed by two leaves containing an acephalous explanation of various calendar units (*lustra, indictio,* the year, the months,[15] and the kalends, nones, and ides). The explanations of these terms are closely related to parallel discussions in John of Sacrobosco's *Computus ecclesiasticus*, from which Daniel derived his presentation of leap year, dominical letters, ways of defining the day, and so on.[16]

The third astronomical insert (ff. 214v–215r) serves as a kind of explanatory note to a list of the zodiacal signs on f. 100r in Book 2, accurately cited by its old folio number: "Os we haue in þe 2 boke, þe 85 lef, of þe 12 sygnis, þe 1 syngne is Aries" (f. 214v). The new material explains the names of the twelve signs in terms of the weather or solar motion at their different times of year. Like the insert on calendar terms, this text is closely related to passages in Sacrobosco's *Computus* or some similar work.[17] Given Daniel's own debt to Sacrobosco, whom he calls "þe Maistere of þe Compote" (R 2.6.272), and that he repeatedly explains medical and scientific terms etymologically, one must at least wonder if these supplementary texts on months, signs, and so on also originated from Daniel's pen but never made it into the main beta tradition. Or perhaps they are the work of someone who recognised Daniel's calendric source material and was inspired to graft in a few more useful digressions on time and the stars.

Taking Egerton 1624 as a whole, it appears that its added materials may have been seen as enhancements to the central uroscopic treatise, supplements dealing with doctor-patient interactions, herbal terminology, astronomy and the calendar, bloodletting and plague, measurement, an alternative learned description of urinary contents, and the navigational aid of a detailed index. Whether the additions were the work of one or more contributors, they would have made the volume even more useful to medical readers.

## IV. Extracts and Abridgements of Individual Books

Four "heirs" to the *Liber Uricrisiarum* consist of long excerpts from one or more of the books in the original work: an unabridged extract from the Lacteus and Karopos chapters in Book 2, which breaks off incomplete near the end of Karopos (London, British Library, Sloane MS 1088, ff. 61r–93v [s. xv]); an unabridged copy of Book 1 and about half of Book 2 (London, Royal College of Physicians, MS 356, ff. 1r–64v [s. xv[in]]), which appears to have been deliberately truncated after the astronomical digression in Lacteus; an abridged version of Book 2 (Oxford, Bodleian Library, MS Rawlinson D.1221, ff. 50r–62v [s. xv]); and an abridged version of Book 3 plus excerpts on crisis and astronomy from Book 2, in the sibling texts in London, British Library, Sloane MS 2527 (ff. 178r–196v, 198v–201v [s. xv]) and London, British Library, Sloane MS 134 (ff. 1r–3v, 4v–20v [s. xv]). A fifth offshoot of Daniel's work that can be placed in this category is John Arderon's commentary on Gilles de Corbeil (Glasgow, University Library, MS Hunter 328, ff. 1r–44v [s. xv[4/4]], and Manchester, John Rylands University Library, MS Eng. 1310, ff. 1r–21r [s. xvi[in]]), which excerpts and embeds descriptive material and diagnostic signs from *Liber Uricrisiarum* books 2 and 3 in Arderon's comments on individual colours and contents.[18]

*London, British Library, Sloane MS 1088*

The text of the Lacteus and Karopos excerpt in Sloane 1088 (Sd) is an unabridged copy of the beta version of those chapters, beginning with the qualities of the planets and the *rota celi* diagram (= Book 2.33, f. 83v, in Oxford, Bodleian Library, MS Ashmole 1404 [1400–25], the best text of the beta version),[19] and continuing to near the end of the material on Karopos-coloured urine (= Book 2.45, f. 106r in Ashmole). The text matches that of Ashmole 1404 (A) closely, including a complete list of physiological signs linked to the planets, correspondences between the planets and metals, and the long "fortunes of men" section on nativities.[20] The most striking difference between Sloane 1088 and the majority of beta texts is that Sloane 1088 employs the alpha version's chapter numbering system for Book 2, with single chapters assigned to each colour or colour-pair (e.g., Rufus/Subrufus) rather than several shorter chapters for each colour. Although the excerpt begins partway into the

Lacteus chapter, and ends shortly before the end of the Karopos chapter, an explicit/incipit between the two chapters makes the numbering clear: "Explicit 6 cap. de lactea vrina. Incipit 7 c. de colore karepos." Cross-references to other chapters are also based on the alpha numbering, referring to the chapters on Blo (lead-coloured) and White urine as the third and fourth chapters, instead of using chapter numbers from seven to fourteen (Blo) and fifteen to twenty-four (White). This combination of alpha chapter numbering with a beta text is most likely a deliberate scribal reversion to the older and simpler chapter structure while retaining the revised text, perhaps because of the frequent errors and omissions in the chapter numbering of beta witnesses – what we might think of as "scribe-proofing" the chapter numbers.

The Sloane 1088 excerpt is atelous, breaking off incomplete shortly before the end of the Karopos chapter. The last quire of the excerpt is wanting its final leaf, which would have been sufficient to finish the chapter. The surviving excerpt may be close to its originally intended extent, which would suggest an interest in the astronomical, astrological, and anatomical digressions in these chapters of the *Liber Uricrisiarum*, along with a respect for the original text or an unwillingness to spend time abridging that text.

*London, Royal College of Physicians, MS 356*

Royal College of Physicians, MS 356 (P) contains all of Book 1 and Book 2 through to the end of the astronomical digression under the colour Lacteus, concluding with correspondences between planets and metals and a final "Explicit liber" beneath the text. A full copy of the beta version of the text up to that point, it has relatively few chapter headings or numbers, but those that do remain correspond in position to the beta chapter structure. Internal cross-references also reflect the many-chaptered beta numbering. The breakpoint occurs just before some of the beta texts (AG6SdSb) offer a further digression on nativities, and it seems possible that the scribe or compiler simply grew impatient with the non-uroscopic material in the treatise and deliberately stopped copying.

*Oxford, Bodleian Library, MS Rawlinson D.1221*

This manuscript (Ra) is a medical miscellany containing Latin and English texts, including several academic uroscopies in verse and prose, glossed in both Latin and English; remedy texts and a regimen by seasons; humoral treatises; and various short medical notes. The uroscopies include a series of *regule* titled "Contenta de vrinis extracta ex dictis Egidii" in the explicit (1r–4v); Gilles de Corbeil's *Carmen de urinis*, glossed in Latin (5r–8v, colours; 12r–14v, contents); *Urina rufa significat bonam dispositionem* (9r–10r); *Omnis urina est colamentum sanguinis* (10r–v); Latin verses *De .19. coloribus vrine*, with English glosses (15r); a passage mainly on urines of death organised by colour, attributed in the explicit to Gord' (Bernard de Gordon; 15r–16r); the Standard Commentary on Gilles's *Carmen de urinis*, with extensive marginal notes, mainly in Latin but occasionally in English (17r–44v; *inc.* "Liber iste quem legendum proponimus"); several components of the *Dome of Uryne* compendium (47v–49v); the Twenty Jordan Series (50r–62v, upper margins); and the abridged version of the *LU*, alpha version, Book 2 (50r–62v, main text).

The texts in the manuscript are written in similar secretary scripts, though the ink varies somewhat in colour and texts may have been added over an extended period of time. Marginal notes are mostly in smaller scripts, but may be by the same writer(s) as the main texts. The manuscript may be an anthology of medical texts made by a university-trained practitioner, comfortable in both Latin and English, and finding useful texts and making annotations in both languages.

What interested the compiler of Rawlinson D.1221 in Daniel's work were the urinary colours in Book 2. He omits most of the non-uroscopic digressions, including the astronomical and calendric portion of the Lacteus chapter, the anatomical section of the Karopos chapter, and a lengthy case history also in Karopos, plus the general discussion of colour in chapter 1. However, he retains (in condensed forms) the explanation of critical days in the chapter on Black urine; some of Daniel's etymological explanations; and some of his catalogues and differentiations of diseases, humours, and other medical topics. The compiler has a strong interest in diagnostic rules, numbering and emphasizing specific uroscopic *regule* with marginal headings (*prima regula, 2a regula*, etc.). This interest in diagnosis may explain the addition of the Twenty Jordan Series (minus its series of twenty medicines) to the margins of the text, matched to the appropriate colour in the *LU*, as that short treatise gives concise lists of various diseases signified by particular colours.[21]

Besides the wholesale deletions of digressive passages, the compiler significantly condenses Daniel's prose by omitting synonyms and glosses, modifiers, repeated nouns (occasionally replaced by pronouns if necessary), qualifying or explanatory comments, cross-references and most citations of authorities, and many etymologies and shorter theoretical observations. Thanks to these condensations and the longer deletions, the Rawlinson copy reduces Daniel's Book 2 text to about 20 per cent of its original length, with reduction results for individual chapters ranging

from 8.6 per cent for Lacteus (due mainly to dropping the long astro-calendric digression) to about 33 per cent for the Rufus/Subrufus chapter.

*London, British Library, Sloane MS 134 and Sloane MS 2527*

These two manuscripts contain a condensed version of Book 3 in the *Liber
Uricrisiarum*, including the final chapter on the "Rules of Isaac" (a translation of *particula* 10 in Isaac Israeli's *Liber de urinis*); the section on critical days from Book 2.2 on Black urine; the section on fevers from Book
2.3 on Blo or Lividus urine, with small additions from Book 2.2 (*lente*
fever) and 2.6 (planetic or erratic fever); and in Sloane 134 only, the digression on astronomy and the calendar from Book 2.6 on Lacteus urine.
The abridgement of Book 3 in Sloane 134 (ff. 1r–3v) is acephalous and
atelous, with only a few lines of Book 3 preceding the "Rules of Isaac"
and breaking off in the "Rules" for Black urine; on the other hand, Sloane
134 does contain the full excerpts on critical days and fevers (ff. 4v–10v)
and astronomy and the calendar (ff. 10v–20v). Sloane 2527 has all of Book
3 and the "Rules of Isaac" (ff. 178r–196v) plus the full critical days and
fevers excerpts (ff. 198v–201v), but it omits the astro-calendric passage.
    Where the two texts overlap, they are textually so close that they
must descend from a common archetype. Sloane 2527 may even be a
direct copy of the original unmutilated text of Sloane 134.[22] I will therefore treat the two witnesses as a single text comprising four separate
excerpts, citing the more complete Sloane 2527 (Se) for the first three,
and Sloane 134 (Sf) for the fourth.
    Comparisons of the excerpts from Book 2 with other versions reveal
that these passages are drawn from the "proto-alpha" version of the
text found in two fifteenth-century codices: Cambridge, Gonville and
Caius College, MS 180/213 and Oxford, Bodleian Library, MS e Musaeo
116 (G3M6; as Harvey observes in chapter 4, the proto-alpha text runs
through Book 2.6, at the end of which the two manuscripts are grafted
onto a beta text). The most noteworthy parallel is the date given for
the year that "we be nohw ['now'] in" in the astronomical digression:
alpha witnesses like London, British Library, Royal MS 17.D.i (ca. 1400)
specify the year as 1378, beta witnesses omit the specific date entirely,
but Sloane 134 and the Caius and Bodleian manuscripts all give 1377
as the year. Another major correspondence also occurs in the astronomical digression in those three witnesses: the transposition of two long
passages, one on the planetary and stellar spheres and the other on
the planetary houses and the governance of the body by the zodiacal
signs, reversing their order in the main alpha version. Smaller verbal
correspondences with proto-alpha G3M6, contrasting with other forms

of the alpha version, occur throughout all three excerpts from Book 2 in
SeSf, still visible despite the abridgements that reduce those excerpts by
anywhere from a quarter to a third of their original proto-alpha lengths.

In the abridgement of Book 3, Sloane 2527 (Se) and Sloane 134 (Sf)
may derive from a beta version of the *Liber Uricrisiarum*, and more precisely to the beta witnesses AG6 EW, rather than the beta star group
M6G3 CfCgHB.[23]

The condensed excerpts of the *Liber Uricrisiarum* in Sloane 2527/134
suggest a compiler/editor who was interested in the more "reliable"
diagnostic indicators given by the contents of urine[24] and some of the
non-uroscopic set pieces that provide larger conceptual frameworks for
medical practice: critical days, types of fevers, astronomy. Like most of
Daniel's adapters, he reduces the general prolixity of his source, but his
cuts are not as draconian as those in some other adaptations; in Book 3,
the overall reduction is about half the original length, while the Book 2
excerpts, as indicated above, range in size from about 65 per cent to 75
per cent of their originals.

### John Arderon, *Commentary on Gilles de Corbeil*

This remarkable text,[25] written in the early fifteenth century, presents the
colours and contents of urine by quoting the appropriate Latin lines of
Gilles de Corbeil's *Carmen de urinis*,[26] followed by brief explanations of
the colour or content and a series of diagnostic signs and their meaning, with attributions of the individual signs to a wide range of learned
authorities: Isaac, Gilles, Avicenna, Theophilus, Gilbertus Anglicus, Bernard de Gordon, and at least as many others. Interestingly, a preliminary
examination of the text reveals that quite a few of the signs also appear in
the *Liber Uricrisiarum*, often with very similar language, though Daniel's
name appears nowhere in the commentary. The author also embeds the
text of the Twenty Jordan Series, illustrated by uncoloured flasks and including the remedies associated with each colour, in the colours section
of his treatise, and appends two small segments of the *Dome of Uryne*
(on substance and on signs of death) and excerpts from another signs-
of-death uroscopy ("Urine Troubly with Clouds") at the end of the text.

Arderon may have felt that a contemporary English compiler of
learned uroscopic materials did not merit citation by name, or that he
was justified in attaching the names of Daniel's own sources (at least
as he understood them) to the signs, but I have not yet been able to
undertake the lengthy task of source-identification required to make
such determinations one way or the other. With the recent appearance
of Javier Calle-Martín's edition of the text,[27] it should now be possible

to work out more clearly which signs are closely paralleled in Daniel, which are not, and whether there is any pattern to Arderon's selection of and attributions for the Danielian signs.

## V. Adaptations of the Full *Liber Uricrisiarum*

Four adaptations of the *Liber Uricrisiarum* preserve content from the entire work, albeit at strikingly differing levels of condensation. The shortest of these adaptations was quite successful in its own right, with multiple copies, while the other three may have been one-off productions, though the last achieved wider distribution by virtue of its appearance in print in or around 1527.

*Seventeen-Chapter Abridgement*

The Seventeen-Chapter Abridgement of the *Liber Uricrisiarum*, first identified by Kari Anne Rand Schmidt,[28] was the most popular and possibly the earliest adaptation of Daniel's work, surviving in three complete stand-alone copies (G5SiL6), one complete copy embedded in a longer medical compendium probably written before 1413 (G7), and two fragments in truncated versions of that compendium (T2W7).[29] It is also one of the most drastic condensations of the original, especially in books 2 and 3. Book 1 is cut to about 24 per cent of the original word-length, while books 2 and 3 are reduced to a mere 7 to 8 per cent of the source. Summed across the whole, the entire Seventeen-Chapter Abridgement is only about a tenth as long as the alpha version of the *Liber Uricrisiarum*.[30]

Among the radical omissions in the Abridgement are the sections on critical days, fevers, astronomy and the calendar, and anatomy, from the chapters on Black, Blo, Lacteus, and Karopos urines. Also omitted are cross-references, etymologies, definitions, many synonyms, and catalogues of maladies and other medical categories. Book 1.1 and 1.2 are combined into a single chapter; all of Book 3 is jammed into a single final chapter. Complex discussions are often significantly simplified, such as Daniel's treatment of the seemingly paradoxical qualities of children's urine in *Liber Uricrisiarum* 1.4.

Unlike most of the other adaptations of Daniel, the Seventeen-Chapter Abridgement goes beyond merely deleting material, adjusting grammar and syntax as needed, and occasionally adding words or brief phrases. Instead, its author often remodels Daniel's language and sometimes even alters the symptoms or diagnoses being described in individual signs, strategies of local revision that may have been partly necessitated by the dramatic shortenings of the text in this version.

The popularity of the Seventeen-Chapter Abridgement can no doubt be attributed to its brevity and perhaps its earliness, but three longer adaptations of the full *Liber Uricrisiarum* also survive, two in manuscript, with interesting reorganizations of Daniel's text, and the third printed ca. 1527.

## London, British Library, Sloane MS 2196

The source text for the fifteenth-century manuscript Sloane 2196 (ff. 3r–42v; Sg) appears to have been a beta text, based on its use of the phrase "Isaac the noble Jew" instead of simply "Isaac" to refer to Isaac Judaeus, a feature of the later version of Daniel's text. Another legacy of the beta tradition is a much-abridged discussion of leprosy at the end of the Rubeus chapter. The reviser omits several longer digressions, including most of the physiology of digestion and urine production in Book 1, the astro-calendric material in the Lacteus chapters and the anatomy passage in the Karopos chapters (1.3–5, 2.30–6, and 2.41–4 in the Ashmole 1404 chapter numbering). He retains several digressions with more immediate diagnostic relevance, but moves them forward into his own first book, thereby creating something like a general introduction to the more specialised diagnostic information in the colours and contents books; in the process, he also significantly rearranges the chapters in Book 1 itself (for details, see Appendix 2, p. 126 below).

This thorough-going revision of Book 1, using material from multiple locations in both Books 1 and 2, shows a deep knowledge of the *Liber Uricrisiarum* itself and a deliberate rethinking of Daniel's Book 1 organization. The first five chapters in the revised Book 1 focus on generalities about the digestions and humours, then non-uroscopic prognostic signs, and finally the complexions. Only after laying this groundwork does the reviser turn to urine itself, drawing mainly but not entirely on the opening chapters of the *Liber Uricrisiarum*. Books 2 and 3 are then free to focus more sharply on the colours (in fourteen chapters, like the alpha chapter structure) and contents (planned for nineteen chapters, though breaking off incomplete at the beginning of 3.16, on Motes/*attomi*, at the end of a quire; one more quire would probably have sufficed to complete the text).

The Sloane 2196 adapter is relatively vigorous in his abridgements: although he preserves some Book 2 digressions by moving them to Book 1, his treatise is still the third-most condensed version of the *LU*, after the Seventeen-Chapter Abridgement and Rawlinson D.1221, averaging out to about 30.5 per cent of the original. Interestingly, he seems to have rethought some of his deletions in the Book 1 chapters on Conditions for Inspecting Urines, as he adds back material from two of those conditions in the last chapter of his Book 1. He was clearly a careful reader of Daniel's original, who wanted to retain much of Daniel's medical-theoretical context, but to locate it all in one easy-to-find position at the start of the text.

## The Book of Narborough

Markedly longer than Sloane 2196, though broadly analogous in adaptive strategy, is the uroscopic and therapeutic treatise in New Haven, Yale Medical School, Cushing-Whitney Library, MS 45 (Y), ff. 2r–94v, titled *The Book of Narborough* in eVK2.[31] The treatise contains four books, three on uroscopy and a fourth given the title "Passionary" in several cross-references. Although a scribal colophon dates the manuscript to 1551, the Narborough text is internally dated to 1442 (f. 9v); it is missing leaves at the beginning and end of the text, as well as a few internal folios, but much of the original remains. Judging by an old foliation system, in which lost text and leaves correspond to gaps in the folio-numbers, approximately 85 per cent of the treatise's three uroscopic books survive, and perhaps 40 per cent or more of its fourth, therapeutic book.

The most significant change that Narborough makes to the *Liber Uricrisiarum* is his addition of the Passionary, described as "this fourth boke" (f. 66r). The Passionary is a *practica* in the usual head-to-toe order, describing ailments and their treatment (covering headache to epilepsy in the ten surviving chapters). Although the book is incomplete, the cross-references to it throughout the text show that a full range of chapters was planned, on topics that included *colica passio*, "womb flux," the stone, fevers, gout, consumption, and so on. None of this remedy material is in Daniel, nor is it organised under herbal headings like Daniel's herbal manual.[32] Neither is the Passionary a version of Gilbertus Anglicus's *Compendium Medicine*, though its content is broadly parallel, as it is with most medieval *practicae*.[33] More work will be required to determine whether it has a single main source like the three uroscopy books or is a compilation that may be original with Narborough.[34]

Setting aside the Passionary, Narborough's broad handling of Daniel's text is characterised by several clearly intentional strategies. Most obviously, he abridges, both in large chunks and at the sentence and phrase level. Based on transcripts made by Mari-Liisa Varila and by E. Ruth Harvey (to both of whom I am deeply indebted), the surviving parts of books 1 to 3 in the *Book of Narborough* are approximately 60 per cent as long as the corresponding books and chapters in the *Liber Uricrisiarum*, maybe a little less. Some of Narborough's larger deletions include Daniel's case histories, several conditions to be considered in

examining urine, many etymological explanations, and various repeti-
tive or overly theoretical passages.

The adaptation also transfers several of the long non-uroscopic digressions from Daniel's Book 2 to Narborough's Book 1. The anatomical discussions in the chapters on Blo and Karopos urine are interwoven with
Daniel's Book 1 chapters on the physiology of digestion and excretion to
yield Narborough's Book 1.3. A long passage on critical days moves from
the chapter on Black urine to become Narborough's Book 1.6, and Daniel's astronomical and calendric detour in the colour Lacteus is almost
completely replaced by a new, significantly shorter,[35] and more formulaic
chapter on astromedicine that serves as Book 1.5 in the later work.

Narborough based his adaptation on a beta text of the *Liber Uricrisiarum*, judging by the inclusion of leprosy in the Rubeus chapter (now
lost, but still indicated in the surviving index to Book 2); a description
of Isaac Israeli in the chapter on critical days as "the noble phyloso-
pher & phisycion"; and the spelling of Petrus Musandinus's name in
the Rufus/Subrufus chapter in a form much closer to that of the beta
than the alpha version.[36] However, like the adapters of Sloane 1088 and
Sloane 2196, Narborough follows an alpha chapter structure, with corresponding changes of internal cross-references. He also gives readers
more explicit navigational signals – like the Rawlinson D.1221 adapter,
he labels and usually numbers individual uroscopic "rules" for each
colour and content, both in the text and marginal notes (if those are
original with Narborough) and in the index to Book 2 that follows Book
3. Finally, Narborough condenses Daniel's prolixity in familiar ways:
reducing synonym lists and glosses, limiting explanatory comments
and qualifications, and so on.

*Judicial of Urines (ca. 1527)*

Our last text is a printed edition of the *Liber Uricrisiarum*, dated 1527?
in STC2 (no. 14836), which received a slightly modified second printing
later in the same year (14836.3). Titled *The Iudycyall of Vryns* (henceforth
*Judicial*), it may reflect a now-lost manuscript exemplar, or may have
acquired its present form during the process of publication. The colophon suggests that the compiler felt some anxiety about the task he and
the typesetter had undertaken, which may mean the rewriting occurred
close to the time of printing:

> I pray you all that reders be of this present worke to except ['accept'] þe good
> mynde and entencyon of hym that compyled it for as moche as he entended
> the same to be for the comen velt ['common weal(th)'] of peopell / & yf

oyu [*sic*] fynde any thynges in this worke expresseth contrary to the oppe-
nys ['opinions'] of auctours / consyder þat it may be thorow þe defaute
of the wryter or of the setter for that horsse is suere that neuer stumbled[37]
/ and here after yf nede be it shal be corected and also other thynges
very expedyent shall be ther vnto added as shortly as reson shall requere
throuhg [*sic*] godes myght. (f. 63r)

The text is based on an alpha original, with the usual long chapters for
each colour and each content. The reviser has tinkered with the text in
two ways: first, many of the longer digressions are removed, including
the Prologue and the first chapter of Book 1 (with renumbering of subsequent Book 1 chapters and cross-references to them); the critical days
section in Book 2.2 (Black urine); the gynecological material near the end
of Book 2.3 (Blo); the astro-calendric passage in 2.6 (Lacteus); the case history of the man from Stamford in 2.7 (Glaucus); the passage on diagnosis
from sputum in 2.13 (Inopos/Kyanos); and the Rules of Isaac and verse
epilogue at the end of Book 3. These omissions bring the edition down
to about three-quarters the length of its original.[38] On the other hand, the
*Judicial* retains the definitions of fevers and the discussion of pulmonary
diseases in 2.3, as well as the anatomy digression in 2.7 (Karopos).

The second category of revision is a general updating and minor
restyling of language, presumably to match the reviser's vocabulary,
grammar and syntax, and general stylistic preferences. This process
does not appear to have been aimed at condensing the language –
some words and phrases are dropped, but others are added, so that
in chapters where no wholesale cuts occur, the final length may actually be slightly greater than Daniel's (thus, chapter 1.1 in the *Judicial*
is about 105 per cent as long as the corresponding *Liber Uricrisiarum*
chapter 1.2). Many of the recurrent vocabulary substitutions shed light
on words that may have become unfamiliar by the sixteenth century:
*mendement* for *allegeaunce* ("easing"), (*a*)*biden* for *bleven*, *swellyng* for *bol-
nyng*, *caste* for *cacche* ("chase"), *-nes*(*se*) for *-hede*, *mydrefe* for *mydrede*,
*breth* and *wynde* for *onde*, *reason* for *skil*, *bladder* for *vesie*, *euyll* for *wicked*,
and *amendyng*, *bredyng* (!), and *wastyng* (!) for *warisshing*.

Other changes include replacing pronouns with their noun referents;
dropping some internal cross-references; and occasionally altering
word order or syntax in minor ways. On top of the longer omissions,
occasional cuts of a sentence or a paragraph can be found, but are relatively uncommon, especially in comparison with other adaptations we
have seen. The overall goal seems to have been improved uroscopic
focus rather than abridgement, with more generous criteria for the retention of ancillary medical material.

## Conclusions

The survival of some twenty manuscripts containing (or likely originally containing) the complete *Liber Uricrisiarum* demonstrates that
many readers of the treatise wanted the whole work and were not
daunted by its size. However, no adaptation of Daniel's magnum opus
expands its uroscopic content – like *Paradise Lost*, "none ever wished
it longer" – and some condense it strenuously. The moves towards
shorter length and sharper focus no doubt reflect a desire for a more
manageable text, but they may also imply a diffusion of general medical knowledge as vernacular medical texts multiplied, reducing the
need for Daniel's definitions and explanations and his often encyclopaedic digressions on non-uroscopic topics.

What the adapters were aiming at naturally varied, but certain recur-
ring *desiderata* can be inferred from the surviving witnesses: some users
found the astro-calendric material of intrinsic interest (Sloane 5, Pepys
1661, Sloane 134) or worthy of supplementation (Egerton 1624); others
were interested in critical days, with or without accompanying uroscopic signs (Sloane 134/2527, JTSA 2611); the Sloane 1088 reviser may
have wanted astronomical *and* anatomical information, without both-
ering to remove the uroscopic material surrounding those passages in
the Lacteus and Karopos chapters; in Sloane 1721, the sixteenth-century writer of the short summary of *Liber Uricrisiarum* 2.1–2 may simply
have been taking notes on those chapters.

Not surprisingly, the practical diagnostic value of the *Liber Uricrisiarum* was recognised and enhanced in revisions focused solely or
primarily on specific colours or contents (Rawlinson D.1221, Sloane
134/2527, Arderon's Commentary, the Seventeen-Chapter Abridgement). Some revisers clearly wanted to retain theoretical and contex-
tualizing information, but preferred to streamline the books on colours
and contents by moving such passages to Book 1 (Sloane 2196, *Book
of Narborough*), while others accomplished such streamlining by simply jettisoning the digressions from Books 2 and 3 (Seventeen-Chapter
Abridgement, *Judicial of Urines*). Finally – and repeatedly – Daniel's
heirs reduce his cross-references, etymologies, source-citations, double
and triple (and longer) synonym strings, and catalogues of the "spices"
of various medical entities.

Although the full *Liber Uricrisiarum* was copied throughout the fifteenth and into the sixteenth century, with active owner-annotators
into the seventeenth, its late-medieval adaptations show that there was
also a market for condensed versions or for select extracts of non-uroscopic "good bits." Given that full versions also continued to be copied,

it seems likely that the wide dissemination of Daniel's groundbreaking work paved the way for its later adaptations and analogues, when readers and adapters had a better idea of what they wanted in an English uroscopy manual, whether concise or comprehensive.

## APPENDIX 1

### Egerton 1624, f. 218r–v:

incomplete ME translation of Bernard de Gordon, *De urinis*, ch. 26, "De contentis"

| Gilles de Corbeil, *Carmen de urinis* | *Liber Uricrisiarum*, Book 3 | Bernard de Gordon, *De urinis*, ch. 26 (*Lilium medicinae*, Lyon 1574: 809–15) | Egerton contents text |
|---|---|---|---|
| Circulus | Circle | Circulus | Circle |
| Ampulla | Ampulla (Bubbles) | Ampulla | Ampulla |
| Granum | Grains | Grana | Grains |
| Nubecula | Nebula (Cloud, Sky) | Spuma | Spuma |
| Spuma | Spuma (Froth) | Obumbratio (si contentum debeat appellari) | Obumbracio (if it be a content) |
| Pus | Sanies (Pus) | Nubecula spiritualis | Rubicula [*error for* Nubecula] spiritualis |
| Pinguedo | Pinguedo (Fat) | Unctuositas | Unctuositas |
| Chymus | Humor Crudus (Raw Humor) | Minuta quasi stillantia | Minuta ?succulancia (*prob. error for* sintillancia)[39] |
| Sanguis | Blood | Sanies & virulentia | Sanies Virulenta |
| Arena | Arena (Gravel) | Pinguedo | Pinguedo |
| Pilus | Pili (Hairs) | Humor crudus | Humor Crudus |
| Furfura | Furfura (Bran) | Sanguis | Sanguis (*text ends incomplete in Sanguis*) |
| Crimnoides | Crinoides | Arenae | |
| Squamae | Squamae (Scales) | Pili | |
| Partes Atomosae | Atthomi (Motes) | Furfurea | |
| Sperma | Sperma (Sperm) | Squamosa seu petaloidalia | |
| Cinis | Cineres (Ashes) | Crimnoidalia | |
| Sedimen | Ypostasis | Alba minuta rotunda | |

## APPENDIX 2

### Sloane 2196: Book 1 chapters and sources

| Sloane 2196, Book 1, chapter and topic: | *Liber Uricrisiarum* source chapter (beta and alpha parallels): |
|---|---|
| 1.1: Of the three digestions and their purgations; seats of the humours, humoral correspondences with cerebral quadrants, day-quarters, seasons | 1.3, 1.5, 2.25, 2.30, 1.10 (= alpha 1.3, 2.4, 2.6, 1.4), Generation of Urine, White Urine, Milky Urine, Conditions of Inspecting Urine |
| 1.2: Good and bad prognostic signs (force of nature, breath, pulse, face, faeces) | 2.6 (= alpha 2.2), Black Urine |
| 1.3: Sputum as prognostic sign | 2.76 (= alpha 2.13), Inopos/Kyanos Urine |
| 1.4: Critical days | 2.4 (= alpha 2.2), Black Urine |
| 1.5: Complexions | 1.10 (= alpha 1.4), Conditions of Inspecting Urine (Kynde) |
| 1.6: Meaning of the word "urine"; regions of body and of urinal | 1.1 (= alpha 1.1), On the Word "Urine"; 2.41–2.45 (= alpha 2.7), Karopos Urine |
| 1.7: Causes of limited and excess urine | 2.50 (= alpha 2.8), Pallidus/Subpallidus Urine |
| 1.8: Twenty conditions in judgment of urine | 1.6–1.18 (= alpha 1.4), Conditions of Inspecting Urine |
| 1.9: General rules on the significance of urine; influence of environment and food; changes in urine after collection | 1.19, 1.13, 1.7 (= alpha 1.4), Conditions of Inspecting Urine (end; Diet/Regimen; How Often) |

NOTES

1  These manuscripts are listed in Table 1 of Harvey, Tavormina, and Star's edition of the *Liber Uricrisiarum* (University of Toronto Press, 2020), pp. 23–5. One manuscript (Br, possibly a beta or beta star text), unseen and now in private hands, could not be included in Harvey's analysis in chapter 4 above.

2  For a list of the most common Middle English uroscopies, see M. Teresa Tavormina, "Uroscopy in Middle English: A Guide to the Texts and Manuscripts," *Studies in Medieval and Renaissance History* ser. 3, 11 (2014): 1–154, at 127–8 (Appendix C). Research for this chapter has led me to identify adaptations of Daniel's text slightly differently than I did in 2014.

3  Two dimensions of Daniel's legacy are not treated here, though they would repay further study: first, marginal annotations by later owners or other readers of the *Liber Uricrisiarum*, such as the bibliophile-physician Philemon Holland (Cf: Cambridge, University Library, MS Ff.2.6), the

medical book collector and rector of Minchinhampton, Gloucs., Henry Fowler (G: Gloucester, Cathedral Library, MS 19), and possibly others; second, a systematic analysis of scribal "translation" patterns in rephrasing Daniel's less familiar vocabulary and morphology over the century and a half between the *Liber Uricrisiarum*'s original composition/revision ca. 1377–1382 and its appearance in print ca. 1527.

4   Including but not limited to a long insertion on leprosy at the end of the chapters on Rubeus and Subrubeus urine; at least two additional case histories; and material on eclipses, climates, planetary physiognomy, and (in some beta witnesses) astrological nativities in the astronomical digression in Book 2. For more detail on these and other beta revisions, see Harvey above, pp. 87–107.

5   Both the incipit and the explicit of this text (ff. 1r, 83v) identify Daniel as the author. The Latin version contains some 43,000-plus words, in contrast to about 116,600 words in the alpha version and the still greater length of the beta version.

6   On the *hereos* addition, see Jake Walsh Morrissey, "Anxious Love and Disordered Urine: The Englishing of *Amor Hereos* in Henry Daniel's *Liber uricrisiarum*," *Chaucer Review* 49.2 (2014): 161–83.

7   Chaucer's *Astrolabe*, which survives in about the same number of manuscripts as the full or originally full copies of the *Liber Uricrisiarum*, boasts only one near-contemporary reference, made by Lydgate in his bibliographic *homage* to Chaucer in the *Fall of Princes*. See Larry D. Benson, ed., *The Riverside Chaucer* (Boston: Houghton Mifflin, 1987), 1092. References to Bartholomaeus Anglicus's *On the Properties of Things* are not uncommon in Middle English scientific prose (Daniel himself has many such citations in his herbal), but probably were meant as pointers to the Latin text rather than Trevisa's translation. See also Peter Murray Jones's chapter in this volume, "Henry Daniel and His Medical Contemporaries in England," 63–83.

8   For a single-manuscript edition of this text, see Javier Calle-Martín and Jesús Romero Barranco, "The Middle English Version of *The Book of Nativities* in London, Wellcome Library, MS Wellcome 411, ff. 9v–18v," *Analecta Malacitana* 36.1–2 (2013): 307–46. As the editors note, the text is a version of a treatise found in multiple manuscripts, frequently accompanying the *Wise Book of Philosophy and Astronomy* (308–9); it is also known as the *Book of Destinary*, the *Book of Fortunes*, and *Book of Fates*. The text and its Latin source(s) and analogues are marked by significant levels of variation in organization and some content, but do appear to have a common underlying origin. Some version of the treatise may also lie at the heart of the nativities digression in the beta version of the *Liber Uricrisiarum* (in Ashmole 1404, Gonville & Caius 376/596, and Sloane 1088; and with significant

modifications in Sloane 1101). Aside from Wellcome 411, none of the copies of the *Book of Nativities (Destinary)* that I have examined (about a dozen of the twenty-plus known Middle English copies) includes the citations of the *Liber (Boke of) Vricrosiarum.*

9   For other manuscripts containing parts of this compendium, including the uroscopic section, see Tavormina, "Uroscopy in Middle English" (2014), 47–9 (item 6.3, *Ten Cold Ten Hot*). For a recent edition of *Ten Cold Ten Hot,* see M. Teresa Tavormina, ed., *The Dome of Uryne: A Reading Edition of Nine Middle English Uroscopies,* EETS o.s. 354 (Oxford: Oxford University Press, 2019), 25–30. Copies of the compendium without the uroscopic material occur in manuscripts such as New Haven, Yale Medical School, Cushing-Whitney Library, MS 47; Cambridge, Gonville and Caius College, MS 457/395; London, Wellcome Library, MS 8004. The mid-sixteenth century *Boke of Knowledge of Thynges Vnknowen* (London: Robert Wyer, 1554, 1556; STC2 11930.7, 11931) incorporates several components from the Sloane 213 compendium, including the uroscopic section.

10   The beta version drops the reference to the current date. Given the s. xv date of the manuscript, the 1392 date in the text is probably inherited from an exemplar, as Rosamund McKitterick and Richard Beadle point out, but no full extant copies of the *Liber Uricrisiarum* have 1392 in their leap-year discussion. Or it may simply be one of the frequent miscopyings of numerals from the original text. See McKitterick and Beadle, *Catalogue of the Pepys Library at Magdalene College, Cambridge.* Vol. v, part 1: Manuscripts, Medieval (Cambridge: Brewer, 1992), 26.

11   E.g., *-ness* for *-hede; glittering* for *glirond; an Ethiopian* for *a man of Ethiop; naturall* for *kynde; it shewethe* for *it is token of,* and occasional errors like *vanishinge* for *warsshing* "healing, recovery."

12   All calculations of reduction percentages in this chapter are approximate. They are based on computer word counts of transcripts of the texts being compared, but those transcripts contain a few words that are not actually part of the texts in question, such as folio numbers, occasional marginalia, editorial headings, etc. Though not absolutely precise, the percentages still give a reasonable picture of relative degrees of condensation across different adaptations of the *Liber Uricrisiarum.*

13   The *Linguistic Atlas of Late Mediaeval English* (*LALME*; ed. Angus McIntosh, M.L. Samuels, and Michael Benskin; 4 vols. [Aberdeen: Aberdeen University Press, 1986]) identifies Hand A (16r–43r) with Ely (1:109). *LALME* groups the other three English hands in the *Liber Uricrisiarum* under the general label "NME" (northern Middle English).

14   Lori Jones has examined the poem and image in "Bubo Men/Pest-Aderlaßmann? Repurposing Fifteenth- and Sixteenth-Century Therapeutic Anatomical Illustrations for the Plague," forthcoming in *Death and Disease*

*in the Medieval and Early Modern World: Perspectives from Across the Mediter-ranean and Beyond*, ed. Lori Jones and Nükhet Varlik (Woodbridge, Suffolk: York Medieval Press). I am most grateful to Professor Jones for sharing her chapter with me in advance of publication. For the text of the poem, see R.H. Bowers, ed. "A Middle English Mnemonic Plague Tract," *Southern Folklore Quarterly* 20 (1956): 118–25.

15 In a further act of supplementation, the names of the corresponding He-brew months are added in a later hand in the margins on ff. 126v–127r.

16 John of Sacrobosco, *Libellus de sphaera: accessit eiusdem autoris Computus ecclesiasticus* ... (Wittenberg: Petrus Seitz, 1543), sigs. B7r–C1r (months), C4r–C5r (kalends, nones, ides), H1v–H3r (*lustrum, indictio*). For a digitised manuscript copy of the *Computus*, ca. 1300, from British Library, Harley MS 3647, ff. 33v–54v, see http://www.bl.uk/manuscripts/FullDisplay. aspx?ref=Harley_MS_3647.

17 *Computus ecclesiasticus*, sigs. C1v–C3v.

18 *John Arderon's* De judiciis urinarum: *A Middle English Commentary on Giles of Corbeil's* Carmen de urinis *in Glasgow University Library, MS Hunter 328 and Manchester University Library, MS Rylands Eng. 1310*, edited by Javier Calle-Martín, Exeter Medieval Texts and Studies (Liverpool: Liverpool University Press, 2020). Arderon is not to be confused with John Arderne, the Anglo-Latin surgical writer of the fourteenth century (Tavormina, "Uroscopy in Middle English" [2014], 99n89).

19 Ashmole puts the diagram a few folios earlier, in ch. 2.30, f. 77r, and sim-ply refers back to it and describes its content in ch. 2.33, f. 83r et seq.

20 The fortunes of men passage appears only in Ashmole 1404, Gonville and Caius 376/596, and Sloane 1088; the full list of physiognomic effects of the planets and the planets/metals correspondences occur in those three man-uscripts and Royal College of Physicians 356. The beta witnesses Egerton 1624 and Wellcome 225 break off at precisely the same point in the physi-ognomy passage (midway through Sol), omitting the planets/metals and fortunes of men before returning to the end of the Lacteus chapters (2.38 in the Ashmole numbering). London, British Library, Sloane MS 1101 (ca. 1450), also a beta text, contains a different version of the fortunes of men passage. The alpha version contains none of these passages.

21 M. Teresa Tavormina, ed., "The Twenty-Jordan Series: An Illustrated Mid-dle English Uroscopy Text." *ANQ* 18.3 (2005): 40–64.

22 The beginning of a marginal note at the bottom of Sloane 134, f. 1r, is in-corporated in Sloane 2527, f. 193r (mid-page), following the last words of the main text on f. 1r of Sloane 134, and then cancelled as the Sloane 2527 scribe apparently recognised that it was not part of the primary text.

23 In the verses listing urinary contents at the end of 3.1, Se AG6EW use the phrases *partes athomose* and *spiritus alta petens* and give the verses in their

correct order, in contrast to the same phrases (but misordered verses) in beta star (M6G3 CfCgHB) or the phrases *necnon atthomique* and *(spiritus) ypostasis octodecem* (with correctly ordered verses) in the alpha tradition (RM7 SaScGT).

24   Cf. Gilles de Corbeil, *Carmen de urinis* 208–11: "The form of colour more often deceives the physician and judgement of the substance frequently betrays his trust; in the contents, there is a firm law, a sure discernment, a constant rule of judgement, and true faith" (in *L'Urologie et les médecins urologues dans la médecine ancienne: Gilles de Corbeil, sa vie, ses oeuvres, son poème des urines*, ed. Camille Vieillard [Paris: Rudeval, 1903], 288; my trans.). Later uroscopic writers and commentators, including Daniel, regularly re-emphasise the point.

25   On the rarity of Middle English medical texts that can be classified as commentaries, see Irma Taavitsainen, "Transferring Classical Discourse Conventions into the Vernacular," in *Medical and Scientific Writing in Late Medieval English,* ed. Taavitsainen and Päivi Pahta (Cambridge: Cambridge University Press, 2004), 37–72 at 51–5.

26   The Rylands copy omits the quotations from Gilles and the Latin Prologue to the work.

27   I am grateful to Professor Calle-Martín for sharing a draft of his edition with me prior to publication, enabling me to make these preliminary observations about the Arderon commentary.

28   Kari Anne Rand Schmidt, *Manuscripts in the Library of Gonville and Caius College, Cambridge.* Index of Middle English Prose, Handlist 17 (Cambridge: Brewer, 2001), 45, 66. The Seventeen-Chapter Abridgement has been edited by Tom A. Johannessen, "The *Liber Uricrisiarum* in Gonville and Caius College, Cambridge, MS 336/725" (MA thesis, University of Oslo, 2005). Available online at https://www.duo.uio.no/handle/10852/25409.

29   For manuscript details, see Tavormina, "Uroscopy in Middle English" (2014), 90–1. The medical compendium was compiled by one "Austyn" for his "dere gossip Thomas Plawdon citiseyn & barbour of london" (Gonville and Caius College MS 176/97, 39). Plawdon is usually identified with the London barber-surgeon Thomas Plouden whose 1413 will survives; assuming that identification is correct, the constituent parts of the compendium – including the Seventeen Chapter Abridgement – must date to the early fifteenth century or before. See Linda E. Voigts and Michael R. McVaugh, *A Latin Technical Phlebotomy and Its Middle English Translation,* Transactions of the American Philosophical Society 74.2 (Philadelphia: American Philosophical Society, 1984), 15 and 15n46.

30   The degree of condensation in the Seventeen-Chapter Abridgement and the reviser's penchant for rewriting and compressing Daniel's language

make it difficult to be sure whether the reviser's source was an alpha or beta text, but there are no obvious signs of the beta version in the abridgement as it stands.

31   The title derives from several appearances of the phrase "quod Narborough" at the ends of individual books of the treatise. The name could be scribal, rather than authorial, but Henry Fowler, the seventeenth-century owner of the Gloucester Cathedral Library copy of the *LU*, whose extensive marginalia accurately cross-reference points in Daniel with parallels in "Narburgh" some ten times, takes the name as authorial and even dates the author to 1464 (Glouc. Cath. Lib., MS 19, f. 37r).

There is a very short extract from the *Book of Narborough* in New York, Jewish Theological Seminary of America, MS 2611 (Jt), ff. 1r–4r, consisting solely of Narborough's chapter on critical days (1.6).

32   Daniel explicitly excludes therapeutic content from the *Liber Uricrisiarum* in his Prologue, promising to treat such matters in another work (possibly his herbal) if his health and superiors allow. On Daniel's plans for works beyond the *Liber Uricrisiarum*, see E. Ruth Harvey, "Medicine and Science in Chaucer's Day," in *The Oxford Handbook of Chaucer*, ed. Suzanne Conklin Akbari and James Simpson (Oxford: Oxford University Press, 2020), 440–55; Harvey, *The Faithful Messenger: Urine and Uroscopy in the Middle Ages*, unpublished study, chap. 5, 43–5 (personal communication).

33   For the long history of the *practica* genre in medieval medicine, see Luke Demaitre, *Medieval Medicine: The Art of Healing, from Head to Toe* (Santa Barbara, CA: Praeger, 2013), 1–33; for representative texts in the genre, see Demaitre's chronology of collated manuals and Bibliography of Sources (325–7 and 333–5).

34   According to Fowler's marginalia, Narborough was a Franciscan friar; Jones has demonstrated the impulse among English friars to create useful and often open-ended medical compilations in such works as the *Tabula Medicine*. See Peter Jones, "The '*Tabula medicine*': An Evolving Encyclopedia," in *English Manuscript Studies 1100–1700*. Vol. 14: *Regional Manuscripts 1200–1700*, ed. A.S.G. Edwards (London: British Library, 2008), 60–85; Jones, "Mediating Collective Experience: The *Tabula Medicine* (1416–1425) as a Handbook for Medical Practice," in *Between Text and Patient: The Medical Enterprise in Medieval & Early Modern Europe*, Micologus' Library 39, ed. Florence Eliza Glaze and Brian K. Nance (Florence: SISMEL/Edizioni del Galluzzo, 2011), 279–307; and Jones, "Henry Daniel and His Medical Contemporaries in England," 63–83, in this volume. Faye Marie Getz, "Charity, Translation, and the Language of Medical Learning in Medieval England," *Bulletin of the History of Medicine* 64 (1990): 1–17, also notes the involvement of friars in the production of English medical books.

35  About 3,400 words in Narborough's text, compared with approximately 5,530 words in the analogous material in *LU*. I have not identified an exact source for the new chapter, though it is thoroughly conventional in content, similar to such treatments as *The Middle English* Wise Book of Philosophy and Astronomy: *A Parallel-Text Edition*, Middle English Texts 47, ed. Carrie Griffin (Heidelberg: Winter, 2013); treatises on *The Seven Planets* (e.g., Peter Brown, ed. "The Seven Planets," in *Popular and Practical Science of Medieval England*, ed. Lister M. Matheson [East Lansing, MI: Colleagues Press, 1994], 3–21 and María José Carrillo Linares, ed. "The Seven Planets," in *Sex, Aging, and Death in a Medieval Medical Compendium: Trinity College Cambridge MS R.14.52, Its Texts, Language, and Scribe*, ed. M. Teresa Tavormina [Tempe, AZ: Arizona Center for Medieval and Renaissance Studies, 2006], 681–99); Bartholomaeus Anglicus's *De proprietatibus rerum*, Book 8; and many more.

36  "Maister Pers Massander" in Narborough (f. 37v), "Mayster Pers Messendene" in the beta text (Ashmole 1404, f. 120v), "Maistre of þe Mesondeu" in the alpha text (R, 2.10.158).

37  Proverbial: "That horse is sure [var. good] that never stumbled." See Bartlett Jere Whiting, *Proverbs, Sentences, and Proverbial Phrases from English Writings mainly before 1500* (Cambridge, MA: Harvard University Press, 1968), H515.

38  This approximate ratio is based on a twenty-page transcript, whose total word count averages 684 words/page. The total length of the text proper is 127 pages (ff. 1r–63r, including a doubled f. 27), plus a four-page index (ff. 64r–65v), so the approximate count for the whole text is just under 86,900 words, compared with an approximate count of 116,600 in the alpha text.

39  Compare the content at the end of John Arderon's commentary on Gilles's *Carmen de urinis*: "20[th] contenta. Syntilla or Sparklys. Syntylla they ben lyke smale sparklys of fyre and they goon downward. upward in þe mydel regioun þe wech is clepyd þe regi[on] perforat. And it betokenyth þe stomak is full of wyckyd humeris and disposyd to spue. Gordianus." (Hunter 328, f. 44r). *Minuta* "lijk smale greynes ... as it were sparclis of fier" is also added as a content, with similar signification, in the Seventeen-Chapter Abridgement of the *Liber Uricrisiarum* (Gonville and Caius 336/725, f. 94v). Similar awareness of Bernard's alternative contents is found in the Sloane 2196 adaptation, which adds the following comment to the Aegidian content list in Book 3.1: "But Bernard of Gord' puttith therto *obumbracio* and *vnctuositas* but these suffise" (f. 34r).

*Chapter Six*

ᴄᴡ

# "Her ovn self seid me": The Function of Anecdote in Henry Daniel's *Liber Uricrisiarum*

HANNAH BOWER

Storytelling was one of the immediate goals of medieval uroscopy: through prolonged analysis of a patient's urine, the practitioner could extrapolate a beginning, middle, and end, which he or she then pieced together to tell the story of the patient's body.[1] The art of constructing coherent explanatory narratives had long been considered an integral part of medical practice: at the beginning of the Hippocratic *Prognostics*, it is proclaimed: "if [the physician] discover and declare unaided by the side of his patients the present, the past and the future, *and fill in the gaps* in the account given by the sick, he will be the more believed to understand the cases."[2] In the *Liber Uricrisiarum* Henry Daniel understood uroscopy in just these temporal terms: echoing the *Prognostics* and Isidore of Seville's definition of medicine in the *Etymologiae*, Daniel informs his readers that "it bihoueþ him þat schal be a leche for to knowe þinges þat ar passede & wete þinges þat now ar & for to se tofore þinges þat ar for to come."[3] This Boethian omniscience – eliding the figures of God, physician, and all-knowing narrator – can be translated into the past state of the body, its present pathological status, and its future condition.

The rest of Daniel's treatise makes explicit the causal relationship between these temporalities: understanding the past urinary behaviours of the body allowed the practitioner to speculate about *how* and *why* it came to be in its present state of sickness; the act of diagnosis could take place. Similarly, examining the colour, consistency, and structure of the patient's current urine enabled the medical practitioner to foresee – through good and bad tokens – what the fate of that body would be; prognosis could occur. There is a clear ethical imperative within Daniel's exhortation: a man possessing the esteemed medieval virtue of prudence decided on a course of action through careful consideration of past, present, and future circumstances. The prudent physician, Daniel suggests, made practical decisions about patient treatment through the same kind of narrative thinking.[4] Indeed, citing earlier medical thinkers, Daniel writes in Book 1 that to be able to pass judgment upon urine, the physician needs to gather many pieces of information about the patient, including their age, gender, occupation, and their physical and emotional state (1.4.3–11). These are precisely the kinds of information normally required to begin a narrative.

Given this association between uroscopy and narrative, it is ironic that the small number of anecdotal narratives that appear in the *Liber Uricrisiarum* actually *complicate* the physician's ability to tell this medical story – or at least to do so alone, through the predominantly visual act of uroscopy, without a multitude of other voices. Along with the rest of his treatise, Daniel's case narratives have not been extensively studied and they are easy to overlook: there are only four substantial anecdotes in the extant versions of the treatise and three of these just occur in the longer, revised version of the text, referred to as the beta revision in this companion.[5] In itself this is not unusual: the inclusion of such experiential narratives in medical writings was still a sporadic and evolving stylistic feature in the fourteenth century.[6] However, there were some historical and contemporary models available to medical writers, particularly in the realm of surgery: medieval surgical writers such as Roger Frugard, Lanfranc of Milan, and John of Arderne frequently depict themselves triumphing over their rival practitioners by diagnosing or curing an ailment that had previously resisted treatment or categorization.[7] Self-aggrandisement is palpable, along with what Peter Murray Jones recognises as an exemplary function: like sermon exempla, the narratives play out in time the teaching – or doctrine – of medical authorities with apparently real, living protagonists.[8] Daniel's scattered narratives differ from these in that (perhaps because of his status as a friar) he never portrays himself as an active medical practitioner; instead he recalls witnessing other healers at work.[9] Nevertheless, a similar exemplary dynamic is present: the anecdotes often give the reader a chance to test the knowledge they have acquired in the treatise by interpreting the symptoms the narrative presents and correctly anticipating its diagnostic conclusions.

The process by which this takes place, however, is more complex than this summary suggests. As Larry Scanlon argues, the relationship between exemplum and authority is never one of perfect, unproblematic correlation: instead of seeing doctrinal teachings as "completely determining [an exemplum's] outcome," Scanlon contends that such doctrine "can only be apprehended narratively because it is produced narratively, and the manner of its production is as much a theme of [the] story as it is a feature of its structure."[10] In sum, the situating of events in time, the extraction of causal relationships between those events, and the possibility for delay, deferral, and other kinds of narrative manipulations means that the exemplum can never just be paraphrased by its moral; the narrative always contains within it the possibility for events to take an unexpected turn towards a different conclusion. This is highly relevant to Daniel's anecdotes: in many of the examples discussed below, he presents the reader at the beginning of the narrative with healers whose authority and capability are affirmed but, paradoxically, also marked as ambiguous, uncertain, or wondrously inexplicable. The ambiguous healers are also often set in dramatic opposition to academically qualified physicians, some of whom possess impressive academic qualifications or eminent social status.[11] Through careful use of deferral, suspense, and dramatically engaging plot devices reminiscent of more literary writings, Daniel keeps these connotations of uncertainty and inexplicability in play until the end of the narrative (and sometimes beyond). Consequently, the anecdotes' endings – which usually vindicate the ambiguous healers – are set up within the narratives themselves to appear socially, culturally, and dramatically surprising.

In this chapter, I argue that the vindication of these ambiguous figures not only completes a de-centring of inadequate medical authorities but also completes a de-emphasizing of sight – the sense integral to uroscopic analysis.[12] Whilst sight is inevitably privileged in the *Liber Uricrisiarum*'s description of the colours, structures, and visible textures of urine, these anecdotes artfully refocus a reader's attention onto sound: Daniel stresses, quite literally, the importance of hearing a plurality of voices during medical encounters. His anecdotes – restraining any excessive trust in the powers of individual vision – therefore underline that, though it "bihoueþ" a medical practitioner to know past, present, and future, that narrative can only be pieced together and spoken collaboratively through a multitude of *different* stories.

## Medical Anecdotes in Context

Debates over the relative merits of experience and authority have a long history: Galen's second-century recommendation to combine theory with practice and reason with observation was echoed by many medieval writers.[13] One finds this pairing dispersed through all kinds of medical writing: practical handbooks by university-trained physicians and domestic remedy books aimed at lay audiences both cite (albeit to different degrees) the theoretical and therapeutic teachings of Greek or Arabic authorities alongside texts labelled as "experimentum": these were often charms, remedies, and practical healing procedures that could not be explained through predominant humoral theories of the body.[14]

Sometimes, this emphasis on experience led to micro-anecdotes in late-medieval medical texts. For instance, a remedy for leprous skin eruptions copied in a large fifteenth-century collection of recipes ends with the following validation: "for it was proved be þe tapster of þe crowne at ware besyde london þe yere of oure lorde god . millesimo . cccc. iij . score . and iiij . yere."[15] This validating claim contains the seeds of narrative: a central protagonist, a time and place, and an action with a resolution. A slightly more developed fourteenth-century example, which records the remedy itself as a narrative, appears in Henry Daniel's herbal, written after the *Liber Uricrisiarum*:

> We knewe a lady þat with þe ious þerof & hony, brayd togidre smal, & leyd in a clene linene cloth, heleth euery scaldyng & brennyng; & on þe same wise sche dede with pety homelok & hony, & ofte we hulpe þerto.[16]

Alongside plenteous citations of Greek, Arabic, and Latin medical authorities, the herbal is peppered with similar attributions of remedies to lay healers, a few of which indicate Daniel's own involvement in the cultivation and preparation of herbs.[17] This was presumably a less invasive and more acceptable kind of medical assistance for a friar to engage in than the action that Daniel merely observes in the anecdotes of the *Liber Uricrisiarum*. We will see, though, that in both texts Daniel was interested in – and supported – the expertise of lay healers outside the institutions of academic medicine. In Sarah Star's words, Daniel's writings do not portray medicine as a "specialized, exclusive field" but as "a whole network of advisers" which is composed of "lay and expert, men and women" and which is irreducible to "a singular point of view."[18] For Daniel, practice and experience were as important as revered written authorities.

Before the late fourteenth and fifteenth centuries, though, this long-rooted investment in experience had only occasionally moved into a sustained use of narrative in medical writings. This was partly because there was little available ancient precedent for it: Hippocrates's *Epidemics* – containing in-depth narratives of observation – does not seem to have been known or cited by Western medieval writers; Galen's *On Prognosis*, also containing case narratives, was translated into Latin in the fourteenth century but does not seem to have been widely read until the second half of the fifteenth century. Available Arabic texts also offered Western readers few models.[19] The first extensive and accessible body of literature offering anecdotal models more regularly in the Latin

of the revised beta text after a long discussion of the causes and symptoms of four kinds of dropsy. It therefore presents an opportunity for readers to exercise their diagnostic skills. The narrative opens with this vivid description:

> I wiste where a woman was, a worthy wyfe skantely of 30 yere age. Her wombe waxed grete as anne woman with child; she movht not go for grete. As she lay, she waxed as a cow vppon calvyng. She myght not lyg but wyde open. Her buttokys galdyn and dwyned awey. She yete [*var.*: eet] and dranke as alder heylest [*var.*: *add* herte and speche never bettere]. Her navel wex grete as manes faste [*var.*: fest]. Alle grete leches that myght be fowde [*var.*: foundyn] came her to [*var.*: *add* and namely on þat was grettest clerk of Engelond of his degre]. Sum seyd she had taken it through litel company of man [*var.*: þorwȝ þe fawte of þe cumpany of man, and þat was fals, for her mayster was sufficient j-nowȝ, and eek she took gret plente besyden as wol was knowen]; sum through drynke; sum through thought; sum through wycked humores gedered in the body, by cause that she never had child. Ther was noon that seyd what was cause. Thei yoven her drynckes, powdres, and emplastyrs; alle helpe [*or* holpe?] not. What was for to helpe noo man wyste; wheder she shuld dye or skape noo man wyste; an hande dyrste noo man her take. Lyf had she nevor more, but þat she myght not go but lyg.[32]

This opening passage stresses the helplessness of the woman's predicament caused by her immobility, swollen body, and withering muscles: as her "wombe waxed grete," her buttocks "dwyned away." The pregnancy similes also communicate the confusion she presents to an onlooker: the woman's inflated body asks to be interpreted in the standard reproductive framework for understanding female bodies, but – as the "as" of the simile registers – it simultaneously evades that explanatory frame. This confusion is increased by the physicians' inability not only to agree on a diagnosis ("sum seyd [...] sum [...] sum [...]") but also to arrive at a correct one: speaking through an omniscient, third-person narrative voice, Daniel closes down their ruminations with the unequivocal "noon [...] seyd what was cause." This, along with the emphatic and emotionally charged tripartite repetition of "noo man wyste," sets the scene for a traditional triumph narrative and the dramatic intervention of a heroic medical practitioner. At the same time, the present lack of expertise functions as an invitation to readers to exercise their own diagnostic capabilities, with the expectation that the resolution of the narrative will eventually confirm or correct their attempt.

The arrival of the anticipated expertise is soon reported; however it arrives in an ambiguous and somewhat inexplicable form:

> At the laste kame a yong man that welle was knowen but not as a leche, nor semyd noo leche [*var.: add* and skylfully cowde on lechecraft, and ȝit lytyl medlyd þerwith but it were for Goddes love or for good felaschep, for onestly he hadde for to levyn upon]. And anon as he saw her and her vrin [*var.: add* manye gentelys and men of holy chirche and me present,] he seyd that wycke on the liuer & in the lappes and in the pittes of the liuer, and the liuer is vnmyghty for to be deliuered þerof, so thei hangen and clevyn and baggyn þeron, and stuffyn & strangyl the liuer, and it is moseld, wasted, & dropped away, passed the 3 party. And the partyes of the liuer so swelted & molten awey saggyn down in þe body, & þer ston- deth lyke grovndsoppes or dreggys of wyne [*var.:* and alle þe guttis and þe wombe rotyth, and alle þe partes swymmyn þerin and flotyn as a ded doke drenkelyd in water]. And in her body is more then 6 [*var.:* 8] galouns lyke malt water, stynckand as anne broke [*var.:* as careyn]. She myght haue ben holpen by tymes, but alle the lechis in Salarn [*var.: add* ne God be þe comoun cowrs of kynde] kan not cure her now. (f. 64r)

The temporal marker "at the laste" affirms the inexplicability of the man's arrival: he comes after an unexplained delay, with no explicit summons, and from no specific place. This is in contrast to the "grete leches" who are sought out ("fowde"), one of whom has the academic prestige of being the "grettest clerk of Engelond." As well as upsetting the intellectual hierarchies erected at the beginning of the narrative, this new arrival destabilises the capacity of sight to discern, judge, and categorise that, in uroscopic analysis, is so key: instead of ascribing a recognisable social or professional label to the man, Daniel writes that he "semyd noo leche." In some manuscripts, an affirmation of his ca- pacities, sporadic practice, and charitable impulses is then inserted, but this does not fully undo the sense of undefined – and therefore inexpli- cable – difference that Daniel creates around the figure.

This inexplicability also manifests itself in the man's actions: imme- diately after he has problematised the visual capacity of Daniel to cate- gorise him, he demonstrates his own marvellous optical powers: "*anon as he saw her and her vrin* [...] he seyd that wycke on the liuer ... " The judgment is almost instant. There is no description of the colour or tex- ture of the woman's urine (which a reader would expect in a uroscopy treatise).[33] Instead the man is able to see straight inside the woman's body, describing its inner workings. Accordingly, unlike the opening pregnancy similes which underline the opaqueness of the woman's exterior, the similes placed in his mouth in some manuscripts render that body's interior instantly transparent: her rotten and disintegrating organs float inside her "as a ded doke drenkelyd in water." This image, along with the man's comparison in some versions between the smell of the water and "careyn" (carrion), foreshadows his fatal prognosis, rhetorically tying together present and future, as it "behovith" every leech to do.

Vision and uroscopy are thus integral to the narrative and, at the same time, peripheral: because the man possesses inexplicable powers of sight and because there is no description of the woman's urine, a reader is encouraged to attempt diagnosis through other clues, only some of which accord with Daniel's preceding description of the four kinds of dropsy. The swelling of the stomach is a symptom of all types but the description of the buttocks as "dwyned awey" recalls Daniel's claim that, in the fourth and worst type of dropsy, "tympanides," the outer parts of the body are "smale and dwynand awey" (f. 63v). Aside from this precise textual echo, though, there is minimal correlation between the case study and the treatise, which instructs readers to distinguish different types of dropsy through the impressionability of the skin, urine colour, and the outward appearance of facial features (ff. 68r–70r). What is more, the detailed description the man gives of the woman's insides in the anecdote ("wycke on the liver & in the lappes and in the pittes of the liuer") recalls Daniel's description of the third kind of dropsy where he claims that superfluous humours are "sumtyme on þe liuer and among his lappes and in the halkys and in the pyttes of the liuer," f. 62v). The narrative does not, therefore, provide the reader with a straightforward diagnostic exercise even if it does, through the staggered description of symptoms and the deferral of an authoritative diagnosis, create time and textual space for that practice: it is only at the end of the story, after the woman has been cut despite the healer's insistence that such treatment is futile, that this diagnostic ambiguity is finally resolved: "And þis malady he seid was tympanides" (f. 64v).

Instead of providing a straightforward illustration, or exemplum, of authoritative doctrine, Daniel seems more interested here in the cultivation of wonder and the dramatic dynamics of the medical encounter itself. This latter concern is conveyed through an emphasis on voice and speech acts: after the debates of the physicians ("sum seyd [...] sum [...] sum [...] Ther was noon that seyd"), the young medical man is depicted articulating his opinions before affirming them with a promise:

Him was axed if she might be corvyn, for wer she smale she felt her self lyf inow [var.: add she seyde]. He seid, 'Ye, but þat shuld not her helpe [...]

And vppon alle thes thinges and poyntes wold he yevon his [*var:* wald he lay hys hede] to smyte of. (f. 64r)

The mysterious young man who is at once "knowen" and, at the same time, peculiarly unknowable ("he semyd noo leche"), ups the stakes of the medical encounter by swearing that – if his prognosis proves untrue – his head can be cut off. He predicts that even if the fluid is drained from the woman's stomach through surgical incision, the rotting parts of the liver will not come out but instead "brede wormes of a ynche or oþer half ynch long, rede and with blak heddes" inside the stomach (f. 64r). He also predicts that "within litel while afterward she shalle be als fulle of water and als grete wombed as she was before" (f. 64r).

The image of decapitation in the young man's oath is then followed by a gruesome and literal act of cutting. Despite the man's insistence on the futility of surgical intervention, a surgeon arrives to cut open the woman's stomach and drain her abdominal fluid:

Cumeth a cyrurgioun and carveth her a litel above þe leske [*var.: add* þe ryȝt half], & hyld it open nerehande 6 wokes; litel ran, & mikel lyke as [*var.:* lyke lyes] of wyne, saue more swarte; but through þe skyn of her novel as water or liquoure through a thynne cloute, passyng 8 galons lyke malt water, the carvyng alle wey after oon [*var.:* alwey doynge], as I seid.

This shocking event is defined by extremes: the hole in the stomach is open for nearly six weeks and almost eight gallons of fluid are drained from it. Readers do not hear the surgeon's voice; instead, he is defined by actions. That association may reflect the fact that surgeons – to a greater extent than physicians – were often associated with practice over theory, the manual over the cerebral. The surgeon's actions, however, end in failure as the woman's death affirms the young man's fatal prognosis and insistence on the futility of surgical intervention.

So, like the marvellous intruder in *Sir Gawain and the Green Knight* who really does end up having his head removed, the young man depicted in this anecdote enters from an undefined outside, confidently bets his head upon his own assertions, and acquires a partly inexplicable authority. That authority stands largely vindicated at the end of the narrative but there is no mention of any gruesome worms appearing from the stomach, raising questions about the possibility of any individual ever possessing complete prognostic knowledge. Furthermore, the young man's voice is placed within a nexus of other voices that point towards alternative perspectives and different ways of telling

that he waits until "þai were al gone" to commence his regimen. So, although Daniel could have based this turn in events on real-life action, he could also have borrowed the device of overhearing from other narrative models, in order to create room within the anecdote for alternative perspectives.

The means by which the man cures himself are not surprising or controversial: in his later herbal treatise, Daniel advocates the use of bugle to treat jaundice.[36] Such herbal knowledge would have been more accessible to a broader section of the population than much of the detailed academic medical theory which Daniel expounds in the *Liber Uricrisiarum:* herbal knowledge circulated in a wide variety of vernacular prose and verse herbals and through oral communication.[37] Indeed, as already noted, the micro-narratives in Daniel's herbal record people of all professions and statuses – friars, gentlewomen, widows, and songmen – exchanging healing expertise. Although it is not revealed where the man in Daniel's anecdote got his knowledge from, it is obvious that he too was part of a larger network of information-sharing: he acts "as he was taght." What is less clear is why he acts. What spurs him to challenge the physician's prognosis when he, unlike the reader, has no apparent awareness that the colour of his urine is a good omen? The text simply tells readers that he "fast þoght on þat word." This could imply that the man attempted to save himself out of defiant desperation. Alternatively, the man's actions could imply an instinctive knowledge of his own wellness; he would then be a vindicated version of the dropsical woman who mistakenly "felt her self lyf inow."

This mystery remains unresolved and, consequently, the man from Stamford retains a subtle but marvellous inexplicability comparable to that surrounding the young man with superhuman sight who "semyd noo leche." Whilst the tale of the dropsical woman resituates the visual practice of uroscopy within the broader medical encounter by not describing the patient's urine and by reducing the examination process to an "anon," this narrative does so by hinging the dramatic action on sound, not sight: the patient's unexpected sensitivity to the quiet sounds of whispering sensitises *readers* to the different protagonists and voices involved in medical encounters: qualified physicians, lay healers, and patients are, the narrative suggests, all part of a larger web of knowledge and expertise and each possesses their own way of narrating illness. Julie Orlemanski's recent work on the use of medical words and concepts in literary works shows that – by virtue of their narrative form – "poetic narratives could encompass multiple kinds of [medical] causation in their plots and could orchestrate competing discourses within their polyvocal bounds."[38] Daniel's narratives are crafted to be similarly polyvocal: as Star observes of the case studies, Daniel "assembles the various viewpoints as a curious but unobtrusive observer [...] displaying a narratological posture comparable to Chaucer the pilgrim in the *Canterbury Tales*, who [...] ostensibly commits himself to rehearsing their narratives 'as ny as evere he kan' (GP, I.732)."[39]

Daniel's narratives are distinctive, though, for the nimble and economical way in which they underline this multiplicity through displacements of sight by sound. This dynamic is even clearer in another of the case studies that appears in the revised beta text and (in abbreviated form) in a condensed Latin version of Daniel's treatise surviving in just one manuscript.[40] The narrative follows a discussion of *mola matricis*, a lump of flesh that grows within the womb, forcing women to appear "as þei wern with childe."[41] This phenomenon – also described by Daniel as a "wunder gobet" or "wunderlumpe" – was discussed by many ancient and medieval medical writers, apparently functioning as an interpretive challenge and a locus for different explanations.[42] Daniel follows Aristotle's claim that *mola matricis* can be the result of sexual intercourse, but describes the various conditions leading to its creation in more detail.[43] He also claims that the phenomenon can occur *after* conception: if the woman "be myskept as if sche take a sorwe, anger, noye or tene," then her "able seed turnyth and chaungith and lesith þe disposicioun and myȝt þat it is disposyd to, and þer dwellyth stylle and gendrith into a gret gobet of flesch."[44] Daniel then summarises Aristotle's description of a woman who suffered from *mola matricis* for three years before being delivered of a lump of flesh so hard that an iron blade could not cut through it. In the beta text, this narrative encourages Daniel to offer his own anecdotal example:

> Also I knew by a wydowe nerehand of 80 age [*varr.* 60 yer of age, 80 ȝere age] & her husbond eke, and thei wern worthi folke. Which widowe, as alle her neyghburhess told in her absence, she yede with child more then 30 wynter and at certeyne tymes had her throwhis. Her ovn self seid me þat 33 wynter she had gon with child by her mayster, for oder man knew she never, and at every fulle of the mone she had here throughess as woman traueland with child (*var.: add* and sekere sche seyde to every man þat with childe sche was). And thus she toke it: as her yougth her maister shuld out of tovne, and felle that a hovnde sterte vnder the hors belly; the hors aferd sterte, and she faste by, the hors overthrew for ferd and alle þat was in her body overturned and walmed; and alle her lyf she was the wers. And yitt toke she noo hurte ne noo harme to þe syght, and welle she knew þat she had conceyvod late afore. Alle thes foreseid sekeness & mischevys & many mo suffereth the foule wrecchedhed of þe fylthe of oure kynd.[45]

In this shorter anecdote, readers can again practise their diagnostic skills on the symptoms presented but Daniel does not exploit narrative's capacity for deferred resolutions to the extent that he does in the previous two anecdotes. His focus here is instead upon *how* the woman's symptoms are narrated by different people. We move through a series of interpretive frames, all signposted by acts of speech. First, "alle her neyghburhess" tell Daniel "in her absence" that "she yede with child more then 30 wynter and at certeyne tymes had her throwhis." Next, she herself describes her ailment, extending, nuancing, and refining the details in the neighbours' account: "*Her ovn self seid me* þat 33 wynter she had gon with child by her mayster, for oder man knew she never, and at every fulle of the mone she had here throughess as woman traueland with child." The woman's explanation rewrites the neighbours' account with added precision: she does not just experience labour pains at "certeyne tymes" but at every full moon and for thirty-three years, not thirty. She also expresses ambiguity over her body's condition: like the surrounding community, she initially claims that she "had gon with childe," but the simile describing herself "*as* woman traueland with child" (with the "as" underlined in one manuscript) registers the gulf between her own experience and that of a pregnant woman.[46] Finally, her assurance that "oder man knew she never" reads as nervous anticipation of the fact that other individuals may tell her story in ways that cast her as morally deviant. This need to control the stories circulating around her illness is reaffirmed by the clause appearing in some manuscripts: "and sekere sche seyde to every man þat with childe sche was." This simplified narrative presumably attracted fewer questions and judgments than the truth. Through this layering of different voices and narratives, then, Daniel affords readers insight into the female patient's position: she is surrounded by narratives that depict her as a living marvel or as a medical or moral exemplum and she herself must continuously re-articulate the past and present condition of her body.

Intriguingly, though, Daniel not only depicts the woman describing her body but also explaining it. The clause "And thus she toke it" introduces a description of the traumatic horse accident that the woman believes triggered her condition; this explanation recalls Daniel's claim in the preceding discussion that extreme sorrow, stress, and disturbance can turn the seed inside the female body into a case of *mola matricis*. Once again, then, Daniel locates medical expertise in a surprising place: the woman does not need a qualified physician to know what has happened inside her. Like the man of Stamford, she does not know what the colour of her urine signifies and sight is not her primary means of understanding the past and present condition of her body: "And yitt toke she noo hurte ne noo harme *to þe syght*, and welle *she knew* þat she had conceyvod late afore." This implies that her knowledge is more instinctive and again demonstrates that there are many ways to understand and narrate a body's history.

Crucially, though, neither Daniel, the woman, nor any other healer offer a prognosis: the narrative leaves the reader with no conception of what will happen to the woman, how much longer she will endure, or how she might be treated, leaving her suspended instead within an ever-suffering present. Her condition therefore remains somewhat inexplicable and exposes the limitations that deny all human patients and practitioners a perfectly omniscient view of past, present, and future. Daniel underlines these limitations by choosing to end the narrative with a generalising moral statement: "Alle thes forseid sekeness [...] suffereth the foule wrecchedhed of þe fylthe of oure kynd."[47] This statement – which carefully refrains from any particular moral judgment on the woman herself – suspends the *whole* of mankind within a sickly present, the end of which can only be foreseen in, and brought about by, the beginnings of eternal life.

### Reading Urine Blind: The Case of Master Giles

The three anecdotes examined so far all shift the *Liber Uricrisiarum*'s emphasis from vision and uroscopic observation onto the limits of this practice and onto alternative, often aural, forms of medical knowledge. These alternative modes of knowing are exemplified by a great range of people and all of them, the case narratives suggest, have a part to play in the polyvocal narrative of illness. Daniel's shortest anecdote – which appears in both the beta and Latin revisions of the text – initially appears to be the most extreme illustration of this decentralization of vision and uroscopy.[48] The anecdote begins with another figure located outside institutional and socially recognised centres of authority in England:

> I knew a leche of gret name – Maister Gyles by name – that never knev lettur, and dyd many gret dedes. Among Saracenes he seyd he lerned. (Ashmole 1404, f. 21r)

Just like the young man who diagnoses the ailment of the dropsical woman, Master Giles is presented by Daniel as a figure whose authority and expertise could be questioned. Firstly, Daniel confirms that Giles had performed many great feats and his title, "maister," mimics that of university scholars. At the same time, however, Daniel states that Giles was illiterate, explicitly placing him outside the bounds not only of learned medicine but, to borrow Monica Green's phrase, "literate medicine."[49] That would not necessarily have troubled medieval readers, since – as Daniel's citation of diverse laypersons in his herbal indicates – all kinds of people, literate and illiterate, dispensed valued medical advice in the later Middle Ages. Nonetheless, Giles's lack of literacy is a clear signal that he operates outside the affirmed intellectual space of the university.

A similar ambiguity is fostered by Giles's claim that he was trained by "Saracenes," a word often used in Middle English to describe Muslims.[50] Some of the most respected scientific authorities in the later Middle Ages (including Avicenna and Al-Fārābī) were Arabic-speaking and Muslim.[51] Because of this and because of the appeal of the exotic, one frequently finds "Saracen" attributions in English medical texts: indeed, Daniel's own herbal designates particular preparations as deriving from "Saracines."[52] However, because of the word's associations with various kinds of racial and religious otherness, "Saracen" was often ambivalent, potentially signalling prohibited, non-Christian practices.[53] As in the other case studies, Daniel fosters these competing connotations simultaneously, skillfully preventing the reader from confidently "reading" the healing figure presented to them. His technique can be compared with Chaucer's mode of writing estates satire in the General Prologue to the *Canterbury Tales*: as Jill Mann carefully illustrated, Chaucer's originality in the Prologue lies in "making our attitude to the whole description uncertain," by presenting readers with conflicting ways of reading and judging the pilgrims.[54] Although Daniel is not basing his presentation of Master Giles on estates satire, he too artfully encourages readers to juggle multiple character outlines and associations.

After setting these connotations in play, Daniel moves on to describe the main event of the narrative: a test set by a resentful woman, which seems to promise to unravel the mystery of Master Giles's expertise.

A wyfe besyde him had skorne of him, on a tyme fel didcasyd [*var.* discrasid] / she mengyd her watur and her kowes water togeder and sent it him to loke. And or the messynger myght take the vrynal out fro the case, 'Lett be stylle,' quod he, 'go home & sey her that she is with a mayde child, this nyȝht begeten of a preste, and her kow with a flecked calf.' This cowth of alle neyȝhbowrs & fowden soth. I was familiar with the leche & with the wyf, & saw the mayde child & the calf. He was blered & nerehand blynd; & thovgh he ne had ne saw not the watur. Of such manere demyng techeth not this faculte. (f. 21r)

Conduct literature for physicians had long warned about such acts of deception, carried out by patients looking to verify their healer's expertise.[55] The ubiquity of such tales sets this anecdote slightly apart from those already analysed, connecting it to a narrative model with a long textual history even as Daniel roots it in everyday empirical experience by claiming that he knew Master Giles and the woman personally.

The scornful wife's test, however, would not have been difficult for readers of Daniel's treatise to imagine themselves or Master Giles passing: immediately before the anecdote, Daniel gives clear instructions for distinguishing human and animal urine, stating that human urine looks thicker close up and thinner when it is looked at from far away, whilst animal urine inverts these properties.[56] In an unexpected twist, however, Master Giles does not just unravel the wife's deceitful mixing of the urine samples, but also gains the upper hand by telling her something she did not expect to find out: he informs her that both she and her cow are pregnant and describes the parentage of both embryos. Here we approach the limits of uroscopy: in the *Liber Uricrisiarum*, Daniel tells readers how to discern that a woman is pregnant and whether she is carrying a boy or a girl through the colour, consistency, and position of *attomi* (or motes) in the urine (3.16.56–65). However, he claims that this is difficult to do and that the task "begyle[n] most man of þis craft" because "attomye in vryn of woman seyn meny þinges" (3.16.40; 42–3). Master Giles's deductions about the parentage of the embryos are even more remarkable. Daniel categorically states that written texts offer no rules for deducing such knowledge from urine: in the Latin verse epilogue to the *Liber Uricrisiarum*, he writes "Nec scriptura docet sed nec natura docebit/ Si fetus pregnantis presbiteri vel militantis" ("Writing does not teach and nor will nature teach, if the foetus of a pregnant woman is a priest's or a knight's," 3.20.399–400). Depicting such deductions not only as unwritten but also as unnatural, Daniel adds that anyone who claims they are able to know such things is merely "pomposus" (arrogant).

Curiously, though, Master Giles is not presented by Daniel as an arrogant blusterer: Daniel maintains that both he and "alle neyʒhbowrs" could confirm the truth of his predictions. Daniel therefore keeps in play the opposing connotations of familiarity and otherness, knowledge and ignorance, erected around the practitioner at the beginning of the anecdote, choosing not to resolve the ambiguity. Like the healing figures in the other anecdotes, Master Giles also seems somewhat inexplicable: this is not only because he can infer information from urine that neither medical texts nor nature show how to ascertain but also because he does so blind and without even looking at the sample: "He was blered

& nerehand blynd; & thovgh he ne had ne saw not the watur."[57] The emphatic triple negative underlines the total negation of vision that seems to occur in the anecdote. In other narratives, we have seen acts of uroscopic observation marginalised and elided or recontextualised alongside different voices and healing expertise; here, however, that act of seeing is *only* present through its negation. Master Giles must acquire his knowledge by means other than vision. Perhaps an awareness of the "skorne" the woman had for him and a socially acquired knowledge of the nature of her sexual liaisons allowed him to deduce the foetus's likely paternity. Or perhaps he acquired such knowledge through more occult means, such as necromancy. Ultimately, Daniel leaves the means ambiguous within the anecdote. This incomprehensibility is heightened by the fact that Master Giles's methods bring about the cessation of narrative and pedagogic speech: Daniel ends the anecdote by stating "Of such manere demyng techeth not this faculte."

In exposing the limitations of uroscopy, then, Master Giles moves beyond the articulatable realm of medicine into unspecified, unspeakable, and potentially occult or necromantic arts. These are ruled out of bounds and yet Daniel's decision to include the anecdote at all affirms the allure of Master Giles's crystal-clear prophetic vision. That clarity is something medicine might only hunger for: after a series of medicinal remedies in a fifteenth-century manuscript, the following lines appear, apparently adapted from Peter of Spain's thirteenth-century eye treatise *De oculis*: "And who so euer can worche wiþ þes wateris and oylis and askis schuld be namyd more a prophet þan a leche."[58] Here, the sharpened vision of the patient is transferred catachrestically to the physician, who – with his infallible remedies – will always be able to foresee a successful cure. The act of "naming" suggests, however, that the physician's sight can only be re-labelled prophetic; it is not intrinsically so.

Daniel also does not attribute any intrinsic or special powers to physicians: although he does not clarify the nature of Master Giles's unexpected knowledge, and though he does not ever link him explicitly to the occult or demonic, he does indicate that – from his perspective – Master Giles is not entirely a *medical* practitioner, using him to illustrate what is and is not appropriate for "this faculte" to engage in. This suggests that, whilst it "bihoueþ" a physician "to se tofore þinges þat ar for to come," he must see this with the fallible, bodily eyes of humanity rather than through any occult means. Ultimately, then, the narrative ends up reaffirming the importance of sight – albeit in clouded form – within medical encounters. Sight marks the border between the utterable discourse of medicine and that of unspeakable or unteachable methods. It keeps the physician and his enabling, but limited, acts of uroscopic vision within the cacophony of voices and audible web of expertise that Daniel's case studies depict.

## Conclusion

In the *Liber Uricrisiarum*, Daniel often associates negative sounds with ignorant, money-motivated, and deceitful physicians. For instance, in the Latin Prologue to the treatise, he criticises the verbosity and lies of such practitioners; in a Middle English translation, this is rendered as, "he þat biholdeþ wel and parfitely þis boke made in wlgare, [...] shal mowe be a parfite domesman in this crafte [...] if he mysvse noȝt a pompouse lif or bostful, ful of wordes, ful of fables & ful of lesingez" (Pro.64–8). He also anticipates the animalistic "hissingz" (Pro.33) of his detractors and, in Book 2, he characterises "vnwise leches" as "bolde braggers þat stonde in chateryng & in clatering & noght in connyng" (2.12.60–1). In these examples, Daniel portrays the ignorant physician as someone who, failing to engage in careful observation and study, brashly proclaims false tales or "fables." His loud stories – here reduced to unintelligible noise, to "chateryng" and "clatering" – are nothing like the careful mapping of past, present, and future that the *Liber Uricrisiarum* enjoins readers to partake in: much of the treatise suggests that the physician can only tell his story after intense and prolonged looking.

As this chapter has demonstrated, however, the four case studies punctuating the revised beta version of Daniel's work take a slightly different approach to vision and uroscopy: in various ways, they shift attention away from the act of looking so central to the rest of the treatise onto other modes of knowing. Often, Daniel does this by sensitizing the reader to speech and sound; this recreates the polyvocal nature of real medical encounters, whilst functioning symbolically to highlight the range of expertise and perspectives germane to healing processes. Daniel's case studies are unusual in the extent to which they give voice to these varied and alternative perspectives. However, there is synergy here with Michael McVaugh's argument that, from the thirteenth century onwards, uroscopy's role shifted in the bedside rituals that established trust between physician and patient: McVaugh contends that, though uroscopy remained a central diagnostic tool for centuries to come, it was just one aspect of the medical encounter for academically trained physicians.[59] In Daniel's case narratives, uroscopy is similarly recontextualised: it is only one part of healing practices and its limitations are exposed as it is set against alternative modes of sensing, knowing, and healing. Here, the lone "chateryng" of the corrupt and ignorant physician is replaced by overlapping, conversing, and (sometimes) competing voices.

The narratives function, then, as loci where these alternative modes can be explored and affirmed. But they are not wholly at odds with the tone of the rest of the treatise: in the rest of the *Liber Uricrisiarum*, Daniel frequently embarks on lengthy digressions into anatomy, physiology, astronomy, and astrology; he is clear that the skilled healer must place uroscopy within this broader context. Similarly, Daniel maintains that his vernacular treatise is designed to educate those without any formal medical education in the basic principles of that discipline; he views medicine as a practice that does – and should – happen outside the bounds of academia, as well as inside them. This also becomes explicit in the anecdotes, when healers and patients with uncertain or questionable origins, education, and authority offer valuable contributions to the diagnosis or cure of the enigmatic afflictions before them. The anecdotes therefore affirm some of the treatise's fundamental principles, even as they extend, challenge, and complicate others. Their narrative form – and the space this creates for dramatic confrontation, disturbance, and dialogue – allows Daniel to incorporate these different perspectives more easily than he can in the pedagogically oriented treatise.

For Daniel, then, narrative is a way of introducing reflection, uncertainty, and wondrous inexplicability into a teaching text otherwise – and by necessity – concerned with clarity and certainty. The narratives may be few in number but the fact that the majority of them were added into the revised version of the *Liber* reaffirms that they were an important mode of reflection for Daniel: worked back into the treatise, they allowed him, and his readers, to think beyond its claims and in a mode more suited to the contingent, unexpected, and inexplicable.

NOTES

1  I am indebted to Churchill College, Cambridge University for the Junior Research Fellowship that allowed me to complete this chapter. I am also very grateful for the expertise, resources, and transcriptions shared with me by the Henry Daniel project team.
2  For the Greek text and this modern English translation, see *Hippocrates: Volume II*, ed. Jeffrey Henderson and trans. W.H.S. Jones (Cambridge, MA: Harvard University Press, 1923), 6–7.
3  Henry Daniel, *Liber Uricrisiarum: A Reading Edition*, ed. E. Ruth Harvey, M. Teresa Tavormina, and Sarah Star (Toronto: University of Toronto Press, 2020), 2.8.156–8. Subsequent quotations from and references to

the *Liber Uricrisiarum* are cited parenthetically by book, chapter, and line number. See *Isidori Hispalensis Episcopi: Etymologiarvm sive originvm*: Vol. 1: Libros I–X, ed. W.M. Lindsay (Oxford: Oxford University Press, 1911), Bk IV, lines 1–2.

4  On prudence, see John A. Burrow, "The Third Eye of Prudence," in *Medieval Futures: Attitudes to the Future in the Middle Ages,* ed. J.A. Burrow and Ian P. Wei (Woodbridge: Boydell Press, 2000), 37–48; on further connections between prudence and medicine, see Kathryn Crowcroft, "Reconsidering Sense: Towards a Theory of Medieval Preventative Medicine," *Postmedieval: A Journal of Medieval Cultural Studies* 8, no 2 (2017): 162–9.

5  See Sarah Star, "Textual Worlds of Henry Daniel," *Studies in the Age of Chaucer* 40 (2018): 202–3 for a brief but illuminating overview of three of the case studies. See also pp. 98–9 of E. Ruth Harvey's chapter in this companion for an overview of how the anecdotes fit into Daniel's overall style and mode of revision.

6  Nancy Siraisi, *Medicine and the Italian Universities*, 1250–1600 (Leiden: Brill, 2001), 243; Chiara Crisciani, "Histories, Stories, Exempla, and Anecdotes: Michele Savonarola from Latin to Vernacular," in *Historia: Empiricism and Erudition in Early Modern Europe*, ed. Gianna Pomata and Nancy G. Siraisi (Cambridge, MA: MIT Press, 2005), 297–324; Marion Turner, "Illness Narratives in the Later Middle Ages: Arderne, Chaucer and Hoccleve," *Journal of Medieval and Early Modern Studies*, 46, no 1 (2016): 64–5.

7  Studies of these writers' use of narrative include Siraisi, *Medicine and the Italian Universities*, 37–62; Turner, "Illness Narratives," 61–87; Peter Murray Jones, "The Surgeon as Story-Teller," *Poetica (An International Journal of Linguistic-Literary Studies)* 72 (2009): 77–91.

8  Jones, "The Surgeon as Story-Teller," 77–91.

9  On the debates surrounding friars' medical practice, see Peter Murray Jones, "The Survival of the Frater Medicus? English Friars and Alchemy, 1370–1425," *Ambix* 65, no. 3 (2018): 232–49 and Angela Montford, *Health, Sickness, Medicine and the Friars in the Thirteenth and Fourteenth Centuries* (Aldershot: Ashgate, 2004). See also Jones's chapter in the current volume.

10  Larry Scanlon, *Narrative Authority and Power: The Medieval Exemplum and the Chaucerian Tradition* (Cambridge: Cambridge University Press, 1994), 30.

11  Elsewhere in the *Liber Uricrisiarum*, Daniel is highly critical of any kind of physician – whether or not they possess academic qualifications or social rank – who acts with ignorance, pride, and self-interest. See for instance Daniel, *Liber Uricrisiarum*, Pro.37 where Daniel affirms that, unlike other healers, he is not motivated to write the treatise by "cause of lucre of fauour as oþer men doþ"; at 2.12.59–62, he also castigates "vnwise leches" or "dogg-leches" that act "onely for mony wynnyng." For a similar criticism

of "dogg-leches" in the beta version of the text, see Daniel, *Liber Uricrisiarum*, 359, note 60.

12  On the integrity of sight to medieval conceptions of knowledge acquisition, see Suzanne Conklin Akbari, *Seeing through the Veil: Optical Theory and Medieval Allegory* (Toronto: University of Toronto Press, 2004), 3–44.

13  See, for example, John Arderne, *Treatises of Fistula in Ano, Hæmorrhoids, and Clysters*, ed. D'Arcy Power (London: Oxford University Press, 1910), 3.

14  Lea T. Olsan, "Charms and Prayers in Medieval Medical Theory and Practice," *Social History of Medicine* 16 (2003): 343–66; Catherine Rider, *Magic and Impotence in the Middle Ages* (Oxford: Oxford University Press, 2006), 160–85; Peter Murray Jones, "Complexio and Experimentum: Tensions in Late Medieval Medical Practice," in *The Body in Balance: Humoral Medicines in Practice*, ed. Peregrine Horden and Elisabeth Hus (New York: Berghahn Books, 2013), 107–28.

15  Aberystwyth, National Library of Wales, MS 572, f. 4r.

16  London, British Library, Additional MS 27329, f. 55va, transcribed by E. Ruth Harvey.

17  For example, London, British Library, Additional MS 27329, ff. 26va, 81va, 95va. On Daniel's sources, see Star, "Textual Worlds," 191–216.

18  Star, "Textual Worlds," 203, 198.

19  Jones, "The Surgeon as Story-Teller," 78; Siraisi, *Medicine and the Italian Universities*, 243. See also Nancy Siraisi, "Girolamo Cardano and the Art of Medical Narrative," *Journal of the History of Ideas* 52 (1991): 581–602, at 588.

20  On chirurgia, see Siraisi, *Medicine and the Italian Universities*, 37–62; Jones, "The Surgeon as Story-Teller," 77–91. On the attempts to reframe surgery as a *scientia*, see Michael McVaugh, *The Rational Surgery of the Middle Ages* (Tavarnuzze: SISMEL/Edizioni del Galluzzo, 2006).

21  Jones, "The Surgeon as Story-Teller," 79.

22  For example, see London, British Library, Egerton MS 1624, f. 87r and f. 129v; Oxford, Bodleian Library, Ashmole MS 1404, f. 63v.

23  Nancy Siraisi, *Medicine and the Italian Universities*, 226; Julie Orlemanski, *Symptomatic Subjects: Bodies, Medicine, and Causation in the Literature of Late Medieval England* (Pennsylvania: University of Pennsylvania Press, 2019), 38–9, 121–7. For an interesting study of case narratives in a Byzantine uroscopic text, see Petros Bouras-Vallianatos, *Innovation in Byzantine Medicine: The Writings of John Zacharias Aktouarios (c. 1275–c. 1330)* (Oxford, 2020), 69–103.

24  Cited and translated in Monica Green, *Making Women's Medicine Masculine: The Rise of Male Authority in Pre-Modern Gynaecology* (Oxford: Oxford University Press, 2008), 93.

25  Jones, "The Surgeon as Story-Teller," 82–4.

26  Jones, "The Surgeon as Story-Teller," 84.

27  Turner, "Illness Narratives," 64–5.

28  Danielle Jacquart, "Theory, Everyday Practice, and Three Fifteenth-Century Physicians," *Osiris* 6 (1990): 140–61; Crisciani, "Histories, Stories, Exempla," 297–324; Siraisi, *Medicine and the Italian Universities*, 226–52.

29  Jones, "The Surgeon as Story-Teller," 85.

30  For a sustained comparison of Daniel, Arderne, and other contemporary medical writers, see Jones's essay in the present volume.

31  Siraisi, *Medicine and the Italian Universities*, 51–2.

32  Oxford, Bodleian Library, Ashmole MS 1404, f. 63v, transcribed by E. Ruth Harvey. Subsequent quotations from Ashmole 1404 are cited parenthetically by folio number.

33  G.E.R. Lloyd notes that Galen's case narratives in *On Prognosis* also do not include detailed descriptions of the urine Galen examined and pulses he listened to. Lloyd's explanation for this is that Galen was working deductively in the case studies from principles already well established (and therefore not in need of clarification or refinement) in his other treatises. (See G.E.R. Lloyd, "Galen's Un-Hippocratic Case-Histories," in *Galen and the World of Knowledge*, ed. Christopher Gill, Tim Whitmarsh, and John Wilkins [Cambridge: Cambridge University Press, 2009], 115–31.) In contrast, I argue that, in his case narratives, Daniel omits or elides such information in order to create room for uncertainty and alternative expertise.

34  See Matthew Michael, "Secret Talk and Eavesdropping Scenes: Its Literary Effects and Significance in Biblical Narrative," *Vetus Testamentum* 65, no. 1 (2015): 91–113.

35  C.A.M Clarke, "Overhearing Complaint and the Dialectic of Consolation in Chaucer's Verse," *Reading Medieval Studies* 29 (2003): 23.

36  London, British Library, Additional MS 27329, f. 55vb, transcribed by E. Ruth Harvey.

37  See George Keiser, "Vernacular Herbals: A Growth Industry in Late Medieval England," in *Design and Distribution of Late Medieval Manuscripts in England*, ed. Margaret Connolly and Linne R. Mooney (York: York Medieval Press, 2008), 292–307.

38  Orlemanski, *Symptomatic Subjects*, 3.

39  Star, "Textual Worlds," 203.

40  For the Latin, see Glasgow, University Library, MS Hunter 362, ff. 27v–28r.

41  London, British Library, Sloane MS 1101, f. 64v, transcribed by E. Ruth Harvey. I have quoted from this manuscript because the explanation of causes is omitted in Ashmole MS 1404, the copy of the beta text used for the transcription of the case narratives.

42  On this interpretive challenge and its place within literary texts, see Sarah Star, "*Anima Carnis in Sanguine Est*: Blood, Life, and *The King of Tars*," *JEGP*

115, no 4 (2016): 442–62 and Katie L. Walter, "The Form of the Formless: Medieval Taxonomies of Skin, Flesh, and the Human," in *Reading Skin in Medieval Literature and Culture,* ed. Katie L. Walter (New York: Palgrave Macmillan, 2013), 119–39.

43 Star, "*Anima Carnis,*" 446.

44 London, British Library, Sloane MS 1101, f. 64v, transcribed by E. Ruth Harvey. I have quoted from this manuscript because the explanation of causes is omitted in Ashmole MS 1404, the copy of the beta text used for the transcription of the case narratives.

45 Oxford, Bodleian Library, Ashmole MS 1404, f. 59r, transcribed by E. Ruth Harvey.

46 See Oxford, Bodleian Library, Ashmole MS 1404, f. 59r for the underlining.

47 On moral standpoints as the distinguishing feature in modern definitions of medieval historical narrative, see Hayden White, "The Value of Narrativity in the Representation of Reality," *Critical Inquiry* 7, no. 1 (1980): 5–27.

48 For the Latin, see Glasgow, University Library, MS Hunter 362, f. 8v.

49 Green, *Making Women's Medicine Masculine,* 12.

50 See *Middle English Dictionary, Sarasin, n.,* entry 1(a).

51 Though Avicenna was Persian, he wrote in both Persian and Arabic. The texts he did not write in Arabic originally circulated widely in Arabic translation.

52 London, British Library, Additional MS 27329, ff. 115ra, 121ra–b, 134va.

53 See *Middle English Dictionary, Sarasin, n.,* entry 1(b) and 1(c).

54 Jill Mann, *Chaucer and Medieval Estates Satire: The Literature of Social Classes and the General Prologue to The Canterbury Tales* (Cambridge: Cambridge University Press, 1973), 20.

55 See, for example, Henry E. Sigerist, "Bedside Manners in the Middle Ages: The Treatise *De cautelis medicorum* Attributed to Arnald of Villanova," *Quarterly Bulletin of the Northwest University Medical School* 20 (1946): 136–43.

56 On possible sources for this advice, see the Explanatory Note to 1.4.502–7 in the *Liber Uricrisiarum,* 318–19.

57 In the Latin version of the case study, he also does not look at the sample but he is not explicitly blind.

58 Cambridge, University Library, MS Kk.6.33, f. 75v. For a modern English translation of Peter's Latin treatise, see Walter J. Daly and Robert D. Yee, "The Eye Book of Master Peter of Spain – A Glimpse of Diagnosis and Treatment of Eye Disease in the Middle Ages," *Documenta Ophthalmologica* 103 (2001): 136.

59 Michael R. McVaugh, "Bedside Manners in the Middle Ages," *Bulletin of the History of Medicine* 71 (1997): 201–23.

Chapter Seven

༄

# The "almost-Latin" Medical Language of Late Medieval England

SARAH STAR

In the Latin Prologue to his fourteenth-century uroscopy treatise, the *Liber Uricrisiarum*, Henry Daniel describes for his readers the different kinds of terminology comprised in the text proper: *Nec mireris O lector si inveniris me ponere terminus quandoque latinas et quandoque prope latinum quod facio magis brevitatis causa. Quapropter etiam exposito uno termino pro quanto mihi occurrerit non iterum expono eundem.*[1] (Do not be surprised, O reader, if you discover that I sometimes use a Latin term and sometimes an almost-Latin term; the reason is for greater brevity. Wherefore also, when I have explained one word, when it occurs again I will not explain it a second time.) These "almost-Latin" terms are English-Latin hybrids: Latin words that Daniel anglicises and further defines in English, such as "cerebre" for "brain." Terms like these may surprise readers because, despite its Latin title and Prologue, the *Liber Uricrisiarum* itself is written in Middle English; dating from ca. 1375–82, it is the earliest known work of academic medicine written in the language. It survives in thirty-seven manuscript witnesses and two early modern print copies, as E. Ruth Harvey has demonstrated, attesting to its wide circulation and influence in late medieval England.[2] Daniel wrote a Latin Prologue to accompany the English text, and the Prologue too was then translated into English.

Daniel's "almost-Latin" terms exemplify his place in the medical tradition: his treatise as a whole straddles the threshold between Latin and English. He wrote in Latin first; the much expanded English version of the *Liber Uricrisiarum* develops his own shorter Latin treatise, now in Glasgow University Library, MS Hunter 362.[3] He draws on a Latin uroscopic tradition dating back to translations of the Greek classics. But he also diverges from that tradition in his choice of language.[4] Other medical writers living and working in England during the fourteenth century – such as Daniel's better-known contemporary, John Arderne – wrote in Latin.[5] By bringing the renowned science of uroscopy into a new language, Daniel was novel in practice, developing much of the vocabulary needed to express scientific concepts in English. Hence the attention to terminology in the Prologue: readers will encounter many new English words, some of which derive from a specialised Latin vocabulary undergoing its first English vernacularization. In the English Prologue Daniel says he does not claim to write new things, "but that I do it newely."[6] Daniel's novelty is linguistic, stylistic, and lexical, reinventing traditional uroscopy with his new English words.

As much of the previous scholarship on Daniel and his texts have made clear, writing a uroscopical treatise in English during the last quarter of the fourteenth century was novel for several reasons.[7] First, the *Liber Uricrisiarum*, like the herbal, is not a translation of a single Latin authority, as was, for instance, John Trevisa's translation of Bartholomaeus Anglicus's *De proprietatibus rerum*; rather, it is a compilation drawing on multiple sources as well as practical experience. And second, as Daniel himself says in the Prologue, he had neither "redde ne harde" (Pro. 4ra) of this science in English before. The ramifications of the second reason on the development of the English language have yet to be analysed in much detail, and I aim with this chapter to motivate further work on the topic. Since Daniel did not know of any uroscopy written in English, doing so required him to contribute to a budding English technical vocabulary. Many of the words needed to express scientific concepts about the human body had not been written down in English before (though some might have been, and likely were, in use). As I've shown in a lexicographic study of one manuscript containing the *Liber Uricrisiarum*, there are over one thousand English words in Daniel's text that either predate or are contemporary with their earliest records in the *Middle English Dictionary* (*MED*) and *Oxford English Dictionary* (*OED*).[8] The high number of early or "new" English words shows that Daniel was correct to characterise his work as writing "newely," and that his significant contribution to medicine overlaps with a similarly substantial one to the English language.

This chapter demonstrates Daniel's legacy in fifteenth-century literary culture. It complements Tavormina's chapter on "The Heirs of Henry Daniel," exploring some ways that later writers extend Daniel's lead. Unlike Tavormina, though, I locate Daniel's heirs beyond the medical sphere alone, analysing the broader cultural poetics indirectly shaped by his precedent. As I have shown elsewhere, Daniel resembles his literary contemporary, Geoffrey Chaucer, in his narrative techniques, vernacular style, and technical innovation.[9] Like Chaucer,

Daniel provides the first attestation of hundreds of English words, many of them scientific: the names for the signs of the zodiac, the four humours, diseases such as epilepsy. Daniel similarly bears significance beyond his immediate context, resonating with the overtly Chaucerian poetry of John Lydgate. Daniel belongs in studies of late medieval vernacularity, as I argue here, providing a previously unexplored connection for Lydgate's aureate diction.

Daniel's *Liber Uricrisiarum*, as section 1 suggests, is as much a treatise *on* English as *in* English, developing through its "almost-Latin" terms a vernacular style at once mundane and aureate. That style, as I show in section 2, anticipates Lydgate as he deploys his own uroscopic vocabulary in the *Fabula duorum mercatorum*. Lydgate shares with Daniel, as section 3 shows, many "almost-Latin" terms and opens for technical language a privileged place in his aureate poetics.

## Henry Daniel

Daniel embraces his role in developing an English technical vocabulary. Much of the Prologue details the process of vernacularization, Daniel's reasons for undertaking it, and the limitations or possibilities of the English language. After explaining that his colleague, Walter Turner of Keton, put him to "an harde wark" (Pro.9) by asking him to write uroscopy in English, Daniel posits two reasons why it has never been written in English before: "ouþer for the langage is vnsufficiant in itselfe, or for þat we kane it noȝt parfitly" (Pro.18–19). He then argues that an English uroscopy will make the science accessible to "moo men" (Pro.48), states that he has gathered information from various sources and "addede to myne owen þat som auctoures affermeth noȝt" (Pro.56–7), explains that he gives both authoritative science and "diffiniciouns and exposiciouns of termes" (Pro.60), declares that he is not necessarily writing new things, but "þat I do it newely" (Pro.79), and, finally, asks for a specific kind of reader and future compiler.[10] He says:

> Therfor in þis werk I aske euermore a trewe [f. 5ra] reder, I desir a meke herer, I biseke euermore a lele & a benigne correctour, for charite broght me more herto þan hardines. Ouer þat I praie euery writer or compiler of þis, þat he kepe my writing, but if he be of þe langage of annoþer contre. For whie as for þe langage of Englissh tong, as anentz a discrete man & him þat hath þe gift of tunge, trewe & parfite craft of ortographie is taugh in þis bok; he that vnderstondes it noȝt, praie he þat he maye interpretate it, seiþ þe trompe of Criste, i. Seynt Poule. (Pro.86–94)

*Trewe & parfite craft of ortographie is taugh in þis bok.* Rather than trans-
mitting uroscopic science alone, Daniel teaches a new kind of English
language, which he intends for future preservation: "kepe my writing."
His concern for textual posterity resembles Chaucer's scrupulousness
in the epilogue to *Troilus and Criseyde*: "And for ther is so greet diversi-
tee / In English and in wryting of our tonge, / So preye I god that noon
miswryte thee, / Ne thee mismetre for defaute of tonge" (V.1793–6). According to Ralph Hanna III, Chaucer here imagines a new kind of pos-
sessive authorship which, among Middle English writers, only Daniel
anticipated: he too envisions a future for his writing that maintains the
perfection of his orthography.[11] Daniel's orthographic self-consciousness
equally recalls the "right writing" taught by the *Ormulum*. Daniel, like
Orm, combines Latin with English learning, and asks future writers
and compilers to attend the specific form of his spelling, not only the
substance of his thought. He does not share with Orm what Christopher Cannon calls an "eccentric and elaborate" spelling system, but he
maintains a similar commitment to make English a language fit for intellectual communication.[12] The word "ortographie" itself shows Daniel's commitment to vernacular innovation: the earliest record of the
word in the *MED* and *OED* is *a*1460, nearly a century after the *Liber
Uricrisiarum*.[13] Daniel introduces a new English technical vocabulary
while simultaneously introducing the English term for a language system.[14] He may be the first to write the word in English, imagining a
future for his orthography while showing how to spell orthography itself. The *Liber Uricrisiarum* is, for Daniel, a way to incorporate uroscopy
into English medical discourse as well as to develop an English technical vocabulary, a way of communicating "newely" and establishing
himself as an authority both on uroscopy and its burgeoning English
lexicon.

"Ortographie" may also be one of Daniel's "almost-Latin" words. It
appears in the Latin Prologue as *orthographie*, and for Daniel, it probably comes into English without mediation from the French. *Orthographie* also appears in Anglo-Norman texts, but Daniel rarely relies on
their lexicon, preferring Latin as "the langage that is right dere to me."[15]
His hybrid term captures his relation to the existing tradition. Daniel
develops a new English vocabulary, teaching a "trewe & parfite ortographie," but he achieves his pedagogical goal only by incorporating the
resources of the Latin language.

The text proper of the *Liber Uricrisiarum* is full of hybrid terms, including the names for the four qualities: "calidite" (1.4.17), heat, from
*caliditas*; "frigidite" (1.4.17), cold, from *frigiditas*; "siccyte" (1.4.34), dryness, from *siccitas*; and "humydite" (1.4.34), moisture, from *humiditas*.

Daniel uses the Latin words when he wants to denote a pathological quality, different from external heat, cold, dryness, and moisture. They express a distinction in physical condition, and establish for diagnosis a more specialised vocabulary in English. And as promised in the Prologue, once he defines them he continues to use them without explaining them again. One gloss is enough, after which the Latinate word appears normalised as part of a familiar English lexicon. Daniel's "almost-Latin" words reappear in the work of later medical writers and translators. For instance, the *MED* cites the *Liber Uricrisiarum* as the earliest instance of "siccite," with Middle English medical translations of the early fifteenth century following after. For "calidite," "frigidite," and "humydite," however, the earliest uses are attributed to such Middle English translations and Daniel is not mentioned at all.[16] Daniel's "almost-Latin" language expresses concepts fundamental for future diagnosticians. Everything that is "bodely and erþely" (1.4.22–3), after all, is composed of the four qualities. They are vital to uroscopy because "The coloure of vryne is causede principaly of þise 2 qualites: *calidite* and *frigidite*, hete and colde" (1.4.16–17), and the "substaunce, þe body of the vryn, is causede of þise 2 qualites: *siccyte* and *humydite*, dryhed and moisthede" (1.4.33–4). The colour of urine, the topic covered by the entirety of Book 2, is determined by "calidite" and "frigidite," and the substance of urine, the topic covered in Book 3, is determined by "siccyte" and "humydite." The hybrid terms are integral to uroscopy and to medicine in general, and they allow Daniel to maintain his connection to Latin vocabulary while establishing a new one in English.

Daniel usually cultivates an aesthetic of the mundane rather than the aureate. In Book 1, chapter 2, for example, he compares how urine cleanses the blood to how whey is produced from the "cloddres & þe clumpres and þe cruddes" (1.2.19) of milk; and in Book 2, chapter 3, he compares the branching of a vein in the shoulder to a "crokede fork" (2.3.111). These everyday, georgic comparisons seemingly eschew Latinate diction for native language and syntax, and they serve a didactic purpose: Daniel attempts to reach "moo men" by recalling the familiar processes and tools of agriculture. But he equally strives for accessibility by combining English with Latin. Just as the Lord in John Trevisa's *Dialogus inter dominum et clericum* argues that more people will have access to knowledge if texts are written in Latin and in English, Daniel aims to make uroscopy "more openly taghte" (Pro.47) by combining the two languages.[17] He effects the combination, on one level, by writing the treatise in Latin before expanding it in English. But he also does it at the level of the individual word when he writes his Latin-English hybrids.

## John Lydgate

Like Daniel, Lydgate can be called mundane, prolix, and dull. The charge is common and partially justified, but it does not necessitate Lydgate's disparagement. Derek Pearsall argues that prolixity comprises a "deliberately cultivated" aspect of Lydgate's style: the monk was trained in amplification at school and he wrote consciously "according to the accepted canons of taste."[18] Lisa H. Cooper and Andrea Denny-Brown, similarly, reclaim Lydgate's mundanity, valorizing his poetry for its engagement with the world (*mundus*) of medieval material culture; "his verse, once dismissed for both its pedestrian content and mediocre style, is in fact fascinating in its very mundanity."[19] Lydgate's poetry is both mundane and verbose, both commonplace and elaborate. At the level of style, it resembles Daniel's prose. Hanna argues that the *Liber Uricrisiarum*, which consistently spans over a hundred manuscript folios, "cannot be described as attractive to those whose main interest is literary" because of its subject matter.[20] But the relentlessly practical *Liber Uricrisiarum* is, too, both mundane and prolix, commonplace and elaborate: while it teaches a practical subject and compares internal workings of the body to everyday objects, it also ushers in a new technical Latinate vocabulary in English.

Lydgate most clearly resembles Daniel in the habitually overlooked *Fabula duorum mercatorum*. Based on the second tale in the *Disciplina Clericalis*, translated from Arabic into Latin in the twelfth century by Petrus Alfonsi, the Middle English poem represents the development of a perfect friendship.[21] Two merchants, one from Syria, one from Egypt, become best friends from afar. The Syrian merchant visits his friend and there enjoys wonderful hospitality. But he soon falls ill, and his host arranges for doctors to diagnose and treat him. None can offer a cure because he is lovesick and refuses to admit whom he loves: his desired woman is meant to marry the Egyptian merchant, and the guest does not want to betray his friend. He eventually comes clean, his friend unhesitatingly offers him the woman and her dowry, and they get married and move back to Syria. The Egyptian merchant later loses all his wealth and travels to Syria. Preferring death over living on in his misery, he falsely confesses to a murder. His friend sees him in jail and then falsely confesses to take his place. Moved by the merchants' love for each other, the true murderer confesses, saving their lives. The Syrian merchant gives the Egyptian half of his wealth, and the latter returns to Egypt.

Lydgate's version of the fable is, unsurprisingly, longer than it needs to be at 910 lines.[22] But, for the few who have written about it, the poem nevertheless displays Lydgate's stylistic prowess. Pearsall, for instance, lauds it as "a systematic application of high-style rhetoric to a simple exemplum" (202) and an "extraordinary performance" (203). "The story, of course," he writes, "sinks" beneath the weight of Lydgate's digressions, "but as an exercise of style it is superb ... The poem must stand, and stand as a warning against any underestimation of the range of Lydgate's skills" (204). Rather than detracting from the poem, the digressive episodes adorn it with displays of Lydgate's stylistic acumen. So too with Henry Daniel, whose frequent comparisons, fanciful etymologies, strings of synonyms, and digressions (such as a lengthy account of the cosmos, spanning seven folios in the manuscript used as the base text for *A Reading Edition*) demonstrate collectively his vernacular prose style.[23] Far from diminishing the medical material, they represent how Daniel writes that material "newely."

Lydgate digresses in describing the Syrian merchant's illness. Pamela Farvolden echoes Pearsall, describing the medical detail as "bewildering" and stating that Lydgate's use of medical terminology is so profuse that it "threatens at times to derail the poem."[24] Lisa H. Cooper, on the other hand, views the episode as central, arguing that the "significance" of the poem lies in "its depiction of illness both physical and fiscal."[25] The merchant's illness signals other kinds of sicknesses, and symbolises the need for purging in both a medical and economic sense. For Cooper, the poem's medical digression is thus significant insofar as it illuminates the financial, mercantile theme. But the medical details hold importance, I argue, on their own terms, revealing Lydgate's connection to medieval English medicine and linguistic innovation.

Lydgate advertises his debt to uroscopy by evoking medieval physician Gilles de Corbeil (d. early thirteenth century). Gilles, as Faith Wallis explained earlier in this volume, authored the *Carmen de urinis*, a highly influential medical poem ultimately included in the *Articella*, the medical textbook studied by doctors in Paris, Montpellier, Naples, and Salerno throughout the later Middle Ages.[26] After a lengthy description of various fevers, Lydgate writes, "And, yif of colra he take his groundement, / Pure or vnpure, citryn or vitellyne, / Gyles you techith to iuge it by uryne."[27] The only medical writer mentioned by name, Gilles stands for Lydgate as an authority on diagnosis, and uroscopy as the authoritative diagnostic method. Like Gilles, who wrote his uroscopy in verse, Lydgate here melds poetic and medical discourses. Gilles taught uroscopy through the medium of poetry; now Lydgate incorporates uroscopy into his own poem through Gilles's medical-poetic guidance. Lydgate further implies his connection to uroscopy when he explains that the Egyptian merchant gathers doctors to tend to his friend, "To taste his poorys and for to deeme his kynde" (270). The manuscripts, according to Farvolden, differ on the key medical term: does Lydgate intend "poorys," internal channels for urine or other bodily fluids, or "pouce," the pulse?[28] In Lydgate's source the doctors test the patient's pulse, but Farvolden nevertheless leaves the word unemended.[29] Farvolden's choice makes sense in context: "poorys" of the sick were tested by medieval doctors and did determine the patient's "kynde," and Lydgate will later express his debt to the great uroscopy authority, Gilles de Corbeil. By implying here a uroscopic diagnosis, and later naming Gilles explicitly, Lydgate assigns uroscopy a central place in his medical poetics.

Lydgate names Gilles alone, but other uroscopic writers may prove equally relevant. Lydgate may rely, for instance, on the French physician, Bernard de Gordon. Mentioned explicitly in Chaucer's *General Prologue* (434), Bernard describes lovesickness in the *Lilium medicinae* in terms "very close to Lydgate's."[30] Lydgate's language resonates with Daniel as well. Unlike the better-known Bernard, who could have been Lydgate's immediate source, Daniel's connection with Lydgate is indirect. The *Liber Uricrisiarum* was probably not read by Lydgate himself, but it codified an English technical vocabulary that later reappears in his *Fabula duorum mercatorum*.

## A Shared Language

Of the many hundreds of medical terms in the *Liber Uricrisiarum* that either predate or are contemporary with their earliest attestations in the *MED* and *OED*, several also appear in Lydgate's *Fabula duorum mercatorum*, in the work of various Middle English poets, including Chaucer, Gower, and Langland, and in later English medical translations, such as Trevisa's translation of *De proprietatibus rerum* (1398) or the Middle English translation of Guy de Chauliac's *Grande Chirurgie* (a1425). They include: frenesye (346); disese (220, 767); accesse (273); quantite (296); qualite (298); myscheef (352, 367); incurable (314); auctour (294); and humour (272, 296, 302, 316).[31] Several words are attested in only the *Liber Uricrisiarum*, other Middle English medial treatises, Lydgate's *Fabula*, and poetry by Chaucer: amor ereos ("lovesickness," 336) and manye ("mania," 344), for instance.[32] Finally, and most importantly, many terms appear in the *Liber Uricrisiarum*, later Middle English medical texts, and in the work of a single Middle English poet: Lydgate. These words appear in late-medieval-English medical texts, Lydgate's poems, and nowhere else, and their written form seems to originate with Daniel. In the *Fabula duorum mercatorum*, they include: frigidite

(324); humidite (313); aquosite (327); unpure (307); citryn (307); vitellyne (307); profoundid (312); etik (309); corrupcioun (337); interpollat (283); effymera (286, 288); sinochus (301); colra (306); tisyk (315); remys (323); oppilat (325); wannysh (326); imagynatif (340); and bollyng (227).[33] The coincidence is striking. Lydgate's uncommon connection with a specialised, technical language and with medical translators suggests his deliberate development of a medical poetics.

The majority of Danielian terms adopted by Lydgate are anglicizations of Latin or, as Daniel would call them, "almost-Latin" words. Daniel anglicises *frigiditas* and *humiditas* as "frigidite" and "humidite," defining them only once before fully integrating them into the treatise as English. The Latinate valence of "wannysh" is subtler: Daniel often adds "-ish" to colour words, using the suffix as an English version of the Latin prefix "sub-." So, *subcitrin* becomes in the *Liber Uricrisiarum* "citrinish." "Wan" is clearly not a Latin word, but the suffix registers Daniel's recognizable process of anglicization, by which specialised vocabulary transforms into a familiar, native idiom. More explicit, however, are "frigidite" and "humidite," as mentioned already, as well as "aquosite" (*aquositus*), "citryn" (*citrinus*), "vitellyne" (*vitellinus*), "etik" (*etica* or *ethisis*), "interpollat" (*interpolata*), "effymera" (*effimerina*), "sinochus" (*sinochus*), "colra" (*colera*), "tisyk" (*pthisica*), and "imagynatif" (*imaginativa*). Lydgate's medical poetics adapts such Latinisms, using terms from a burgeoning vernacular vocabulary that might have been first written down by Daniel. He adorns his English verse with terms that exist on the thresholds of poetry and medicine, English and Latin.

Many of Lydgate's "almost-Latin" terms appear in close proximity to each other, in the stanzas outlining the merchant's illness. But Lydgate does not simply describe what the illness *is*; he also describes what it *is not* in great detail. Once the doctors arrive and examine the patient, "They seide, certeyn, it was noon of the thre [types of fever], / But yif it were oonly effymora; / For neithir etyk it was ne putrida" (285–7). The poet then uses twenty-eight lines explaining these fevers and their causes, even though the merchant suffers from none of them, except perhaps for "effymora" (and, as it turns out, he doesn't). These four stanzas are certainly digressive – why discuss fevers that the merchant does not have? – but they are significant nonetheless. It is here that Lydgate evokes Gilles and establishes his connection to authoritative uroscopy: "And yif of colra he take his groundement, / Pure or vnpure, citryn or vitellyne, / Gyles you techit to iuge it by vryne." He also showcases his medical knowledge: he knows different kinds of choler exist, he knows their names, he knows what they signify. But he simultaneously highlights his aureate diction, using three almost-Latin terms: "colra," "citryn," and "vitellyne." Derived from *vitellum* (egg yolk), for instance, *vitellyne* describes the consistency of a viscous choler, and has few citations in the *MED*, all from the *Liber Uricrisiarum*, Middle English translation of Chauliac, and the *Fabula*. The digression makes room for Lydgate's experiment with a medical poetics, in which he fuses specialised knowledge with self-consciously elevated diction.

The stanzas on fevers also build towards identifying the illness: "he were falle, for ouht they cowd espye, / For thouht or love into malencolye" (321–2). The diagnosis comes through an examination of physical evidence – from what the doctors "cowd espye" – and so we then hear what it is they saw:

> His vryne was remys, attenuat
> By resoun gendryd of ffrigidite,
> The veyne ryueers, for they wern oppilat,
> It was ful thynne and wannyssh for to see;
> The streihte passage causyd aquosite,
> Withoute substaunce to voyde hym of colour,
> That they dispeired been by his socour.                    (323–9)

Analysing their patient's urine, the doctors judge as Gilles teaches, and put his uroscopic method to practice. Like the doctors, Lydgate learns from Gilles's example, and supplies his description of watery urine in verse. But Lydgate also intersects with Daniel. Several terms in the stanza are first written down in English in the *Liber Uricrisiarum*, and some, such as "frigidite" and "aquosite," are noticeably "almost-Latin." The passage about uroscopy uses terms first used in English in a uroscopy treatise, revealing Lydgate's connection to the tradition as a whole as well as to the project of vernacularization that its English authority, Henry Daniel, ushered in.

As with the digression on fevers, Lydgate combines his medical and stylistic expertise. "Frigidite" and "aquosite," referring to pathological coldness and urinary wateriness, are "almost-Latin" terms that appear only in Lydgate's poetry and medical treatises. But Lydgate also aims for a high style. The *Fabula* is written in rhyme royal, with stanzas of seven lines rhyming ABABBCC. Lydgate ends the second and fifth line of the stanza above with "frigidite" and "aquosite," respectively, using them as rhyme words. Many of the Danielian "almost-Latin" words, in fact, either rhyme with each other or with other, frequently polysyllabic, words: "sinochus" rhymes with "thus"; but "vitellyne" rhymes with "vryne"; "effymora" rhymes with "putrida"; "interpollat" rhymes with "estat"; "imagynatif" rhymes with "estimatiff" and "successyf"; "frenesye" and "manye" rhyme with "malladye." These are not the only polysyllabic words that rhyme with each other in the poem, but their effect is conspicuous: he uses his "almost-Latin" terms, attested only in Daniel and Middle English medical translations, to achieve a more sophisticated sounding rhyme than monosyllables allow. The medical terms increase Lydgate's scientific authority, while enhancing his poetic aureation.

The trend in Lydgate scholarship has long involved documenting and analysing his Chaucerian imitations, and "Lydgate himself invites this kind of reading."[34] He names Chaucer explicitly in the *Troy Book*, the *Life of Our Lady*, the *Fall of Princes*, the *Temple of Glass*, and the *Flower of Curtesye*; and he crafts *The Siege of Thebes* as his own Canterbury tale, complete with a Prologue that places Lydgate himself within Chaucer's frame narrative. Studies of the *Fabula*, less explicitly Chaucerian than the *Siege*, still often rely on comparisons to Chaucer. Pearsall compares it to the *Man of Law's Tale* and *Knight's Tale*; and Farvolden notes that the medical details draw on the *Knight's Tale* and *Troilus and Criseyde*.[35] Some recent scholarship moves away from this pattern and considers Lydgate individually. Cooper, for instance, argues that the "rich fullness" of Lydgate's poetry "comes most clearly into view" "only when we take Lydgate on his own terms, removing him forcibly from the Chaucerian shade in which he himself often tried to stand."[36] Others suggest that Lydgate's "own terms" are themselves Chaucerian, and so a deep understanding of Chaucer and his poetic influence should remain central to studies of Lydgate.[37] The tension, I'm suggesting, points towards the need for a broader analytical scope. Lydgate's verse is undeniably and explicitly Chaucerian, but the *Fabula* and its medical poetics shows that it may also, implicitly, be more than that.

Lydgate's *Fabula* omits explicit reference to Chaucer, but nevertheless imitates his style by using rhyme royal and a polysyllabic lexicon. Scholars since at least Derek Brewer and P.M. Kean have noted that Lydgate models his aureate style on Chaucer even while his poetry distinguishes itself from his predecessor.[38] Cannon explains that aureate diction "came to define the lexical legacy that the fifteenth century understood Chaucer to have bequeathed to it." Polysyllabic borrowings in English, Cannon continues, "are not only the salient feature of Chaucer's high style but precisely the contribution he was understood to make to English by those imitators who actually used his words."[39] When Lydgate and his contemporaries extol Chaucer for making English a literary language worthy of poetry, they are praising in part his polysyllabic lexicon. The aureate diction that Lydgate embellishes in his own poetry defines what Cannon calls Chaucer's high style, and in Lydgate's eyes at least, represents a newly sophisticated English poetry.[40]

I would add that Lydgate's poetic style is Danielian even while it is Chaucerian. Writing about Chaucer's aureate diction, John Norton-Smith argues that technical language, including medical terms, does not count as aureation and should not be considered in studies of it.[41] For Lydgate's aureation, however, technical language seems central. Kean points out that Lydgate associates four images with aureation: "sugar," "balm," "licour," and "dew." He writes:

> As Lydgate uses them, 'balm,' 'licour' and 'dew' all stand for a healing, enlivening, cordial liquid which is distilled either by a plant in the process of its growth, and as the cause of growth, or by a heavenly body as it sheds its influence (also associated with growth) on the earth. Sugar – in 'sugred,' etc. – refers to the sweetness of the plant substances and also to something which is a medicine and preservative in its own right. When we remember that this is also true of Lydgate's central image of gold itself, we can see that this imagery forms a close nexus, linking the ideas of growth, health, vigour, in a totality of meaning which, while Lydgate certainly has style in mind, is more appropriate to the expression of an idea of poetry as a whole and, more particularly, of that relation of style to content which is needed to make an effective statement of the work as a whole.[42]

Lydgate's aureate words all connote healing: "balm" most clearly evokes a medical discourse, but "licour," "dew," and "sugar" have medical connotations as well, referring to methods of healing and restoration.[43] As Kean points out, the medical connotations of these images are "also true of Lydgate's central image of gold itself." The goldenness of aureation is, for Lydgate, intricately linked to ideas of "growth, health, vigour." Kean's observation shows that, despite Norton-Smith's claim that technical language does not contribute to aureation, it is for Lydgate part of the very language that describes aureation. Reading Lydgate "on his own terms" thus includes paying attention to his vernacular technical vocabulary, which he shares with Henry Daniel. His aureation may be modelled explicitly on Chaucer's, but aureation itself evokes a medical discourse that has yet to be fully analysed in Lydgate scholarship and that Henry Daniel helped develop in English.

NOTES

A short version of this chapter was given as a conference paper at the New Chaucer Society in Toronto, 13 July 2018, on the session "Aureation," organised by Nicholas Watson. I'm grateful to Watson for the opportunity to present the paper, to Catherine Sanok for facilitating the ensuing discussion, to the attendees for their helpful questions and comments, and to Christopher Cannon for reading it and commenting on it after the session.

1  Oxford, MS Bodley e Musaeo 116, f. 65v, transcribed by E. Ruth Harvey. The English translation is my own. There are three distinct versions of the Latin Prologue, and these two sentences appear in version 1 only. Version 2 is printed as Appendix 1 in Daniel, *Liber Uricrisiarum: A Reading Edition*, ed. E. Ruth Harvey, M. Teresa Tavormina, and Sarah Star (University of Toronto Press, 2020), 285–8.
2  For an overview of the manuscript families, see E. Ruth Harvey's chapter in this volume, "Textual Layers in the *Liber Uricrisiarum*," 87–107, and Harvey and Tavormina's "Introduction" in *A Reading Edition*, 20–30.
3  Glasgow, Glasgow University Library, MS Hunter 362, ff. 1r–83v.
4  For an overview of the uroscopic tradition from its origins through the twelfth century, see Faith Wallis's chapter in this volume, "Latin Traditions of Uroscopy," 17–37.
5  Peter Murray Jones's chapter in this volume, "Henry Daniel and his Medical Contemporaries in England," 63–83, examines in detail the relationship between Daniel and English authorities such as John Arderne.
6  *Liber Uricrisiarum*, Pro.79. This and all subsequent quotations from the English Prologue and text proper are from Daniel, *Liber Uricrisiarum: A Reading Edition*, ed. Harvey, Tavormina, and Star (2020). Quotations from the Prologue will be cited by line number, while quotations from the text proper will be cited by book, chapter, and line number.
7  In this volume, see Wallis, "Latin Traditions of Uroscopy," 17–37 and Jones, "Henry Daniel and his Medical Contemporaries in England," 63–83. See also Tavormina, "Uroscopy in Middle English: A Guide to the Texts and Manuscripts," *Studies in Medieval and Renaissance History*, 3rd series, 26:11 (2014): 1–154, and Star, "The Textual Worlds of Henry Daniel," *Studies in the Age of Chaucer* 40 (2018): 191–216.
8  See Star, "Henry Daniel, Medieval English Medicine, and Linguistic Innovation: A Lexicographic Study of Huntington MS HM 505," *Huntington Library Quarterly* 81.1 (2018): 63–106. The number of words should not be considered final since this is a study of only one manuscript.
9  Sarah Star, "The Textual Worlds of Henry Daniel" (2018).

10  Daniel claims in the Prologue that "Walter Turnour of Ketoun" (Pro.5), his "belouede felowe in Crist" (Pro.4) asked him to "gadre" (Pro.7) for him "one handeful of flourez of þe domes of vrines, and þat I shulde write þe it shortly and þat in wlgare, i. comune langage" (Pro.7–8). Daniel's argument that writing in the vernacular will make the treatise more widely read can be read through the framework provided by John Trevisa in his *Dialogus inter dominum et clericum*, in which the Lord contends that the widest array of readers can be reached when Latin and English traditions work in tandem. The *Dialogus* is printed in Ronald Waldron, "Trevisa's Original Prefaces on Translation: a Critical Edition," Edward Donald Kennedy, Ronald Waldron, and Joseph S. Wittig, ed., *Medieval English Studies Presented to George Kane* (Suffolk: D.S. Brewer, 1988), 285–99.

11  See Ralph Hanna III, *Pursuing History: Middle English Manuscripts and their Texts* (Stanford: Stanford University Press, 1996), 175.

12  See Christopher Cannon, *The Grounds of English Literature* (Oxford: Oxford University Press, 2004), 82–110, quoted from 84.

13  Both the *MED* and *OED* cite the Middle English verse paraphrase of Flavius Vegetius Renatus, *De re militari* (Cambridge, MS Pembroke 243, a1460) as the earliest attestation, and as one of only two uses prior to the sixteenth century.

14  E. Ruth Harvey and M. Teresa Tavormina believe that the Prologue was translated into English by someone other than Daniel (*Liber Uricrisiarum*, "Introduction," 13). If they are correct, the use of "ortographie" would still signal the significance of the *Liber Uricrisiarum* to the development of the language. Though we could not attribute to Daniel himself the first instance of the term in English, we could still argue for his desire to preserve the language since the passage appears in the Latin Prologue as well.

15  The Anglo-Norman Dictionary also records *ortographie*. Though it appears in the Latin Prologue, it could also be a French loanword rather than an "almost-Latin" term. Since Daniel prioritises Latin as "the langage that forsoth is right dere to me" (Pro.82) and as the language from which much of his material derives, this and other French words were likely, for Daniel, Latin-ish.

16  *MED s.vv.* "siccite" (n.), "calidite" (n.), "frigidite" (n.) (b.), and "humidite" (n.) (1. (b.)).

17  See above, n. 10. The exchange between the Lord and the Clerk is summarised in greater detail by Fiona Somerset, *Clerical Discourse and Lay Audience in Late Medieval England* (Cambridge: Cambridge University Press, 1998), 63–9.

18  Derek Pearsall, *John Lydgate* (London: Routledge and Kegan Paul, 1970), 7 and 8, respectively.

19   Lisa H. Cooper and Andrea Denny-Brown, *Lydgate Matters: Poetry and Material Culture in the Fifteenth Century* (New York: Palgrave Macmillan, 2008), 1.

20   Ralph Hanna III, "Henry Daniel's *Liber Uricrisiarum* (Excerpt)," *Popular and Practical Science of Medieval England*, ed. Lister M. Matheson (East Lansing: Colleagues Press, 1994), 188.

21   The Latin version is printed, with an English translation, in Eberhard Hermes, ed. *The Disciplina Clericalis of Petrus Alfonsi* (London: Routledge and Kegan Paul, 1977).

22   Pearsall writes that the tale "might take up half a page of the *Gesta Romanorum*" in *John Lydgate* (1977), 202.

23   Star, "The Textual Worlds of Henry Daniel" (2018): 191–216.

24   Pamela Farvolden, "Introduction to *Fabula Duorum Mercatorum*," Farvolden, ed., *Lydgate's Fabula Duorum Mercatorum* and *Guy of Warwyk* (Kalamazoo: Medieval Institute Publications, 2016), 7–28, quoted from 15 and 14, respectively.

25   Lisa H. Cooper, "'His guttys wer out shake': Illness and Indigence in Lydgate's *Letter to Gloucester* and *Fabula duorum mercatorum*" *Studies in the Age of Chaucer* 30 (2008): 303–34, quoted from 313.

26   Faith Wallis, "Latin Traditions of Uroscopy," 17–37. For information on the *Articella*, see Thomas F. Glick, Steven John Livesy, and Faith Wallis, ed. *Medieval Science, Technology, and Medicine: An Encyclopedia* (New York: Routledge, 2005), 53–4.

27   This and all subsequent quotations from the poem are from *The Minor Poems of John Lydgate*, ed. H.N. MacCracken (Published by the Early English Text Society, by Humphrey Milford, Oxford University Press, 1910–1934) II: 21. In Farvolden's edition, "colra" appears as "Colre," giving the term a slightly more English appearance.

28   *MED, s.v.,* "pore" (n.(1)), 2.(a).

29   Farvolden, "Explanatory Notes to *Fabula Duorum Mercatorum*" (2016), 62.

30   Farvolden, "Introduction to *Fabula Duorum Mercatorum*" (2016), 15. See also Ethel Seaton, *Sir Richard Roos, c. 1410–1482: Lancastrian Poet* (London: R. Hart-Davis, 1961), 275. Seaton claims that Lydgate's description is "verbally close" to Bernard's and suggests Bernard as a direct source.

31   *MED, s.vv.* frenesie (n.) (a); disese (n.) (4); acces(se (n.) (1.(a)); quantite (n.) (1.(a)); qualite (n.) (3.(a)); meschef (n.) (3); incurable (adj.) (a); auctour (n.) (2.(a)(b)); humour (n.) (3.(a)).

32   *MED, s.vv.* amor ereos (n.); hereos (n.); mania (n.).

33   *MED, s.vv.* frigidite (n.) (b); humidite (n.) (2.(c)); aquosite (n.) (a); unpure (adj.) (a); citrin(e (adj. & n.) (2.(b)); vitellin(e (adj.) (a); profounden (v.) (b); etik (n.(2)) (1.(a)); corrupcioun (n.) (2.(a)); interpolate (adj.) (a); effimera (n. & adj.); sinoch (n.) (a); colre (n.) (1a.) (1c.(a)(b)); tisik(e (n.); remis(se

(adj.) (c); oppilat(e (adj.); wannish (adj.) (b); imaginatif (adj. & n.) (4.(a)); bollinge (ger.) (b).

34  Jeff Espie, "(Un)couth: Chaucer, *The Shepheardes Calender*, and the Forms of Mediation," *Spenser Studies* 31 (2017): 243–71, quoted from 259. Espie argues that Lydgate's lament for Chaucer's death, though not exclusive to his poetry, is "a recognizable characteristic of a Lydgatian mode" (255) and that Lydgate "regularly frames the loss in relation to his own present moment, his own temporal now" (256). Lydgate invites readers to compare him with Chaucer in part by bringing Chaucer into his own poetic and temporal context.

35  Pearsall, *John Lydgate* (1970), 202–4; Farvolden, "Introduction to *Fabula Duorum Mercatorum*" (2016), 13–14 and 16–17.

36  Cooper, "'His guttys wer out shake'" (2008): 313–14.

37  For example, Amanda Walling follows Cooper's prompt, arguing that Lydgate distances himself from his Chaucerian model in *Life of Our Lady* and *Life of Saint Margaret*, in which, she argues, Lydgate's aureation centres on the sanctified female body rather than a patriarchal relationship. See Walling, "Feminizing Aureation in Lydgate's *Life of Our Lady* and *Life of Saint Margaret*," *Neophilologus* 101.2 (2017): 321–36. Pearsall, on the other hand, argues that "Lydgate's career, poem by poem, is a determined attempt to emulate and surpass Chaucer in each of the major poetic genres that Chaucer had attempted" in *John Lydgate* (1970), 47; and Espie, following Pearsall's lead, suggests that the two poets' works are inextricable in "(Un)couth: Chaucer, *The Shepheardes Calender*, and the Forms of Mediation" (2017), though Espie also contests the conventionally patrilineal vocabulary, for which see "Literary Paternity and Narrative Revival: Chaucer's Souls from Spenser to Dryden," *Modern Philology* 114 (2016): 39–58.

38  D.S. Brewer, "The Relationship of Chaucer to the English and European Traditions," *Chaucer and Chaucerians: Critical Studies in Middle English Literature*, ed. D.S. Brewer (London: Nelson, 1966), 1–38; and P.M. Kean, *Chaucer and the Making of English Poetry: The Art of Narrative* (London and Boston: Routledge and Kegan Paul, 1972), II: 210–39. See also Lois A. Ebin, *Illuminator, Makar, Vates: Visions of Poetry in the Fifteenth Century* (Lincoln and London: University of Nebraska Press, 1988), 2–18; and Seth Lerer, *Chaucer and His Readers: Imagining the Author in Late Medieval England* (Princeton, NJ: Princeton University Press, 1993), 22–56.

39  Christopher Cannon, *The Making of Chaucer's English: A Study of Words* (Cambridge: Cambridge University Press, 1998), 153. See also J.D. Burnley, *A Guide to Chaucer's Language* (Norman: University of Oklahoma Press, 1983), 136–9. Cannon goes on to argue that Chaucer's polysyllabic borrowings are not necessarily new and may in fact be quite traditional

"insofar as they *are* borrowings" (153), suggesting that Chaucer's aureation is rooted in tradition if it is based on borrowings alone.

40   Cannon, *The Making of Chaucer's English* (1998), 154, shows that polysyllabic words comprise over a tenth of Chaucer's entire vocabulary, and that polysyllabic rhyme defines his high style.

41   John Norton-Smith, *John Lydgate: Poems* (Oxford: Clarendon Press, 1966), Appendix: Aureate Diction, 194.

42   Kean, *Chaucer and the Making of English Poetry* (1972) II: 231.

43   *MED, s.vv.* "licour" (n.) 3.(b); "deu" (n.) 2; "sugre" (n.) (f.).

# Appendix:
# Content Guide for the *Liber Uricrisiarum:*
# *A Reading Edition*

The content guide for the *Liber Uricrisiarum: A Reading Edition* lists the topics contained in the Prologue, Epilogue, and each chapter of Daniel's treatise. The guide aims to both give readers a picture of the text's entire composition and help readers locate specific topics of interest efficiently.

The chapter titles, provided here in Middle English, come from the internal Table of Contents in London, British Library, Royal MS 17.D.i, which corresponds to lines 105–49 of the Prologue as printed in the edition. The topic descriptions within the chapters are editorial. Daniel may have considered the topics labelled "Digression" as integral to the chapters in which they occur. At least once, however, he acknowledges that he has "gone out of [his] waie, i. a litil fro [his] purpos," while still asserting that he has "noȝt erryd" in so doing (2.6.496).

**Prologue**

Dedication to Walter Turner;

Concern over criticism by hostile readers and modesty tropes;

Value of uroscopy but lack of English texts on the topic;

Sources for the book;

Title of book;

Material benefits of studying uroscopy;

Aristotle on growth of knowledge from earlier works;

Plans for further treatise on remedies if health and religious obedience allow;

Divisions of the book.

## BOOK 1

### Ch. 1: Of significacion (i. of knowyng) of this worde *vrina*

Etymological interpretations of the word *urine*; medicinal uses of urine

### Ch. 2: What vryn is & wherof and how it is made

Definition of urine; comparison of urine to milk and its components whey, butter, cheese, and milk proper; urine as a sieving out or cleansing of impurities in the blood

### Ch. 3: Of generacioun of vryn

Three digestions:

1 in the stomach leading to the intestinal system and solid waste;
2 in the liver, lungs, gall bladder, and spleen generating humours, with the blood sent to the kidneys for cleansing and excretion of waste via the urine;
3 residues of food digested in the solid members of the body to form flesh, sinew, and bone, with waste matter excreted as various bodily substances (e.g., sweat, spittle, earwax, nasal mucus, hair, and raw humours and *ypostasis* in the urine)

Physiology and anatomy of digestive system, cardiovascular system, liver, gall bladder, spleen, urinary system

Diseases affecting the skin: various types of sores, ulcers, and cancers

### Ch. 4: Which þing & how meny bene to be considerede of a leche and how he schulde haue him in demyng

Condition 1: Which it is: The quality, i.e., colour, of urine (see Book 2 for details)

Condition 2: What it is: The substance or body of urine, i.e., density of urine

Condition 3: Which things are therein: Contents in urine (see Book 3 for details)

Condition 4: How much it is: Intensity of colour, quantity of urine

Condition 5: How many times: Frequency of urination, collection, and examination; techniques of examination

Digression: Bladder and other excretory system diseases

Condition 6: Where: Where contents appear in the urine sample; the vessel in which to collect urine; strata of the urine sample; position of vessel with respect to light

Condition 7: When: Time of day for taking sample (for times and frequency of examining, see condition 5)

Condition 8: Age: Age-based differences in urine (caused by age-based complexional differences)

Condition 9: Complexion: Differences based on sanguine, choleric, phlegmatic, and melancholic temperaments; correspondences among elements, prime qualities, humours, complexions; gender-related hot and cold complexions; Latin couplets on the four temperaments, with English translations; relation to the ages of man, in different medical and ecclesiastical systems; relation to seasons of the year, in medical and ecclesiastical systems

Condition 10: Kind: Sex of patient; distinguishing male, female, and animal urines; limitations on determining embrionic temperaments (human) or colours (bovine)

Condition 11: Travail: Activity, study, thought, labour, travel, weariness; also the opposite negative conditions of excess rest and ease

Condition 12: Ire: Anger, sorrow, annoyance, pain, dread, worry, thought and study

Condition 13: Diet: Regimen, general moderation in living, eating, drinking, clothing, work and rest, sleeping and waking; environment, air, terrain, winds; correspondences of compass directions, winds, seasons, humours, elements, ages of man, prime qualities

Condition 14: Busy-ness, Cure: Cares, worries, thoughts that disturb the humours

Condition 15: Hunger or thirst: Excessive fasting, abstinence, lack of food and drink

Condition 16: Moving: Activity, exercise, rest (as discussed in condition 11)

Condition 17: Washing: Bathing in fresh, hot, cold, salt water

Condition 18: Eating: Quality and quantity of food

Condition 19: Drinking: Quality and quantity of drink; colours of drinks (e.g., white wine, red wine); diuretic or styptic effects of drinks

## Ch. 6: *De lacteo colore*, of Mylk-whit colour

Description of colour; causes of the colour; diagnoses based on the colour

Digression: On the seven planets (qualities, "course" or length of orbit, colours, influences on terrestrial life); interspersed with sections on

measurement and divisions of days;

measurement and divisions of zodiacal signs;

calendric information (under Sun, in relation to the year as the Sun's orbital period; includes extensive leap year explanation and calculations of dominical letters, Roman additions and subtraction of days in July, August, February);

Digression: On the Ptolemaic model of universe, including inter-sphere distances and sizes of planets in comparison to the earth; fixed stars, *primum mobile*, empyrean heaven

Digression: Houses of the planets (zodiacal signs where planetary power is greatest); qualities of the planets and signs; governance of the signs over body parts; position of the moon in the signs; hours of the planets

Digression: Distinction and causes *of frigus, rigour*, and *oripilacio* in fevers

## Ch. 7: *De colore karopos*

Description of colour; causes of the colour; diagnoses based on the colour; *Karopos* always thick, while White, Yellow, and Milk-white are thin or thinnish

Digression: Case history of man at Stamford (*Karopos* vs. Yellow diagnoses)

Digression: Descriptions and causes of *colica passio, iliaca passio,* kidney and bladder stones; foods that dispose patients to the stone

Digression: The four regions of the body, and anatomy of those regions

*Membra animata* (head, brain, sensory organs; includes psychological functions of three cells of the brain)

*Membra spiritualia* (respiratory and cardiac systems from epiglottis to diaphragm)

*Membra nutritiva* (stomach, liver, gall bladder, spleen, intestine, membranes around digestive organs)

*Membra generativa* (kidneys, bladder, testicles/ovaries, penis, womb, vulva, clitoris)

Digression: The four regions of the urine and correspondence to regions of the body

*Circulus urine*

*Corpus aereum, regio spiritualis*

The middle of the urine

The *founde* (= *fundus*) or ground of the urine

**Ch. 8: *De pallido colore*, of Pale colour [includes Subpallidus; chapters 9–12 on Citrine through Rubicundus colours likewise include the associated sub-colours]**

Description of colour; causes of the colour; diagnoses based on the colour

Digression: Four kinds of choler (with 2 subkinds for black and green)

Digression: Seven causes of scanty urine; seven causes of copious urine

**Ch. 9: *De citrino colore*, of Citrin colour**

Description of colour; causes of the colour; diagnoses based on the colour

**Ch. 10: *De rufo colore*, i. Rudy colour**

Description of colour; causes of the colour; diagnoses based on the colour

**Ch. 11: *De rubeo colore*, of Rede colour**

Description of the colour; causes of the colour; diagnoses based on the colour

**Ch. 12: *De rubicundo colore*, of Blode-rede colour**

Description of the colour; causes of the colour; diagnoses based on the colour

Digressions: Distinctions between various fevers: *synochus* and its three forms (*homothena, augmastica, epamastica*) and *synocha; causonides, synochides, causon*

**Ch. 13: *De colore ynopos*, i. Swart Rede colour (also includes *kyanos*)**

Description of the colour; causes of the colour; diagnoses based on the colour

Digression: Distinctions between *epatica passio* and pleurisy (apostemes of the liver vs. apostemes of the ribs)

Digression: Diagnostic significance of different kinds of sputum

### Ch. 14: *De ueridi colore,* i. of Grene colour

Description of the colour; causes of the colour; diagnoses based on the colour

## BOOK 3

### Ch. 1: Of 18 contentes of vryn: General discussion

### Ch. 2: *De circulis vrine,* of Cerclez in vryn

Descriptions of Circles (White, Purple, Red, Pale, *Blo*/Leaden, Green, Black, Tremulous); causes and diagnoses

### Ch. 3: *De ampullis,* i. of Burblez in vryn

Descriptions of types of Bubbles (permanent, non-permanent; *tumida, non tumida*); causes and diagnoses

### Ch. 4: *De granis,* i. of Greyns in vryn

Description of Grains; causes and diagnoses

### Ch. 5: *De nebula,* of Cloude of vryn

Description of *Nebula* (*Nubes,* Sky); causes and diagnoses

### Ch. 6: *De spuma vrine,* of Froþ in vryn: Foam

Descriptions of types of Froth (*spuma ventosa, spuma granulosa, spuma continuata, spuma viscosa*); causes and diagnoses

### Ch. 7: *De sanie vrine,* of Quytter in vryn: Pus

Descriptions of types of Pus (based on source in liver, kidneys, or bladder); causes and diagnoses

Distinguishing Pus, Raw Humour, and Ypostasis (see also 3.9)

### Ch. 8: *De pinguedine vrine,* i. of Fatnesse of vryn: Greasiness, oiliness

Description of types of Fatness; (fat urine, oily urine; general Fatness, particular Fatness); causes and diagnoses

### Ch. 9: *De humore crudo,* of Rawe Humour in vryn: Undigested humours

Distinguishing Pus, Raw Humour, and Ypostasis (see also 3.7)

Description of Raw Humour; causes and diagnoses

Five ways to distinguish Raw Humour from Ypostasis

**Ch. 10: *De sanguine vrine*, of Blode in the vryne**

Descriptions of types of Blood in urine (based on sources in bladder, kidneys, liver, or *kilis* vein); causes and diagnoses

**Ch. 11: *De arenis*, i. of Grauel in the vryne: Sandy particulates**

Description of types of Gravel (White, Red, Black); causes and diagnoses

**Ch. 12: *De pilis vrine*, of Heres in the vryne**

Description of types of Hairs (based on source in kidneys or desiccation of humours); causes and diagnoses

**Ch. 13: *De furfuribus*, i. of Scuddes or Brenne in þe vryn**

Description of Bran; causes and diagnoses

**Ch. 14: *De crinoidibus vrine*, of Crepines in vryn**

Description of Crinoids (and distinctions from Bran); causes and diagnoses

**Ch. 15: *De squamis vrine*, of Scales in the vryn**

Description of Scales (and distinctions from Bran and Crinoids); causes and diagnoses

**Ch. 16: *De atthomis vrine*, i. of Motes in the vryn**

Description of Motes; causes and diagnoses (gout in men and women; pregnancy or uterine disease in women)

Gout

Pregnancy

Digressions: General and particular signs of conception; sex of embryo; fertility tests for men and women, causes of infertility in women

**Ch. 17: *De spermate vrine*, of Sperme in the vryn**

Description of Sperm in urine; generation of Sperm (from brain to kidneys to testicles and penis); diagnoses of Sperm appearing in urine or passing involuntarily

**Ch. 18:** *De cineribus vrine*, **of Asshen in vryn**

Description of Ashes in urine; causes and diagnoses

**Ch. 19:** *De ypostasi in vrina*

Definition and five properties of Ypostasis; types of Ypostasis (based on location in sample: *sedimen, eneorima, nephilis*); causes and diagnoses

Colours of Ypostasis (White, Red/Rubea, Subrubea, Livida, Viridis, Nigra)

**Ch. 20: Of general reulez þat Isaac setteþ in þe ende of his bok:** *particula* **10 of Isaac Israeli's** *Liber urinarum* **(sections with following headings):**

Citrine urine; White urine; White and watery urine; Red urine; Rufus urine; Green urine; Black urine; Oily urine; Bright and clear urine; Turbid urine; Ypostasis; Nebula; Urines of women

**Epilogue**

Latin verse indicating general aim of book, limits to what uroscopy can diagnose, dating to 1379

# Works Cited

**Primary Sources**

Agilon, Walter. *Gualteri Agilonis Summa medicinalis*. Studien zur Geschichte der Medizin Beiheft 3, edited by Paul Diepgen. Leipzig: Johann Ambrosius Barth, 1911.

Angeletti, Luciana Rita, Berenice Cavarra, and Valentina Gazzaniga, ed. and trans. *Il De urinis di Teofilo Protospatario: centralità di un segno clinic*. Rome: Casa editrice Università La Sapienza, 2009.

*Alphita*. Edited by Alejandro García González. Florence: SISMEL/Edizioni del Galluzzo, 2008.

Arderne, John. *Treatises of Fistula in Ano, Hæmorrhoids, and Clysters*, edited by D'Arcy Power. London: Oxford University Press, 1910.

Arderon, John. *John Arderon's* De judiciis urinarum: *A Middle English Commentary on Giles of Corbeil's* Carmen de urinis *in Glasgow University Library, MS Hunter 328 and Manchester University Library, MS Rylands Eng. 1310*, edited by Javier Calle-Martín. Exeter Medieval Texts and Studies. Liverpool: Liverpool University Press, 2020.

Avicenna. *Canon*. Lyon: Symphorien Champier, 1522.

Bartholomaeus Anglicus. *Bartholomaeus Anglicus De Proprietatibus Rerum*, Vol. 6 Liber XVII, edited by Iolanda Ventura. Turnhout: Brepols, 2007.

Bernard of Gordon. *Bernardi Gordonii opus, Lilium medicinae inscriptum ... Vni cum aliquot aliis eius libellis*. Lyon, Guliel. Rouillius, 1574.

*The Boke of Knowledge of Thynges Vnknowen*. STC2 11930.7, 11931. London: Robert Wyer, 1554, 1556.

Bowers, R.H., ed. "A Middle English Mnemonic Plague Tract," *Southern Folklore Quarterly* 20 (1956): 118–25.

Brown, Peter, ed. "The Seven Planets." In *Popular and Practical Science of Medieval England*, edited by Lister M. Matheson, 3–21. East Lansing, MI: Colleagues Press, 1994.

Calle-Martín, Javier, and Jesús Romero Barranco, eds. "The Middle English Version of *The Book of Nativities* in London, Wellcome Library, MS Wellcome 411, ff. 9v–18v," *Analecta Malacitana* 36.1–2 (2013): 307–46.

Carrillo Linares, María José, ed. "The Seven Planets." In *Sex, Aging, and Death in a Medieval Medical Compendium: Trinity College Cambridge MS R.14.52, Its Texts, Language, and Scribe*, edited by M. Teresa Tavormina, 681–99. Tempe, AZ: Arizona Center for Medieval and Renaissance Studies, 2006.

Chaucer, Geoffrey. *The Riverside Chaucer*, edited by Larry D. Benson. Boston, MA: Houghton Mifflin, 1987.

Chauliac, Guy de. *Inventarium sive Chirurgia Magna*, edited by Michael R. McVaugh. Leiden: E.J. Brill, 1997.

Daniel, Henry. *A Critical Edition of the Middle English "Liber Uricrisiarum" in Wellcome ms. 225 [microform]*, edited by Joanne Jasin. PhD diss, Ann Arbor, 1983.

– *Liber Uricrisiarum: A Reading Edition*, edited by E. Ruth Harvey, M. Teresa Tavormina, and Sarah Star. Toronto: University of Toronto Press, 2020.

– "The *Liber Uricrisiarum* in Gonville and Caius College, Cambridge, MS 336/725," edited by Tom. A. Johannessen. MA thesis, University of Oslo, 2005. https://www.duo.uio.no/handle/10852/25409.

Gaddesden, John. *Rosa Anglica Practica Medicinae*: Pavia: Fransiscus Girardengus and Johannes Antonius Birreta, 1492.

Gilbertus Anglicus. *Healing and Society in Medieval England: A Middle English Translation of the Pharmaceutical Writings of Gilbertus Anglicus*, edited by Faye Marie Getz. Madison: University of Wisconsin Press, 1991.

Gilles de Corbeil. *Liber de uirtutibus et laudibus compositorum medicaminum*, edited by Mireille Ausécache. Florence: SISMEL/Edizioni del Galluzzo, 2017.

– *Aegidii Corboliensis carmina medica*, edited by Ludwig Choulant. Leipzig: J.B. Hirschfeld, 1826.

Goltz, Dietlinde, ed. *Mittelalterliche Pharmazie und Medizin: dargestellt an Geschichte und Inhalt des Antidotarium Nicolai*. Stuttgart: Wissenschaftliche Verlagsgesellschaft, 1976.

Green, Monica H., ed. and trans. *The Trotula: A Medieval Compendium of Women's Medicine*. Philadelphia, PA: University of Pennsylvania Press, 2001.

Griffin, Carrie, ed., *The Middle English Wise Book of Philosophy and Astronomy: A Parallel-Text Edition*. Middle English Texts 47. Heidelberg: Winter, 2013.

Guy de Chauliac. *Inventarium sive Chirurgia Magna*, edited by Michael R. McVaugh, Leiden: E.J. Brill, 1997.

Henry of Huntingdon. *Anglicanus Ortus: A Verse Herbal of the Twelfth Century*. Edited and translated by Winston Black. Studies and Texts 180. British Writers of the Medieval and Early Modern Period 3. Toronto: Pontifical Institute of Mediaeval Studies; Oxford, Bodleian Library, 2012.

Hippocrates. *Hippocrates: Volume II*. Edited by Jeffrey Henderson and translated by W.H.S. Jones. Cambridge, MA: Harvard University Press, 1923.

Isaac Judaeus. *De urinis* 5, *Omnia opera Ysaac*. Lyon, 1515.

Isidore of Seville. *Isidori Hispalensis Episcopi: Etymologiarvm sive originvm libri XX: Vol. 1: Libros I–X continens*, edited by W.M. Lindsay. Oxford: Oxford University Press, 1911.

John of Sacrobosco. *Libellus de sphaera: accessit eiusdem autoris Computus ecclesiasticus* ... Wittenberg: Petrus Seitz, 1543.

Lydgate, John. *Lydgate's Fabula Duorum Mercatorum* and *Guy of Warwyk*, edited by Pamela Farvolden. Kalamazoo: Medieval Institute Publications, 2016.

– *The Minor Poems of John Lydgate*, edited by H.N. MacCracken. Published by the Early English Text Society, by Humphrey Milford, Oxford University Press, 1910–34.

Macer. *Macer Floridus de Viribus Herbarum una cum Walafridi Strabonis, Othonis Cremonensis et Ioannis Folcz Carminibus similis argumenti* ..., edited by L. Choulant, 1–123. Leipzig: Leopold Voss, 1832.

– *A Middle English Translation of Macer Floridus de Viribus Herbarum*, edited by Gösta Frisk. Uppsala: Almqvist & Wiksells, 1949.

Marbodus Redonensis. *Liber Lapidum. Lapidario*, edited and translated by Maria Esthera Herrera. Paris: Les Belles Lettres, 2005.

– *Macri, De materia medica, libri V*, edited by Ianus Cornarius. Frankfurt: F.C. Egenhalf, 1540.

– *Marbode of Rennes' (1035–1123) De lapidibus*, edited by John M. Riddle and translated by C.W. King. Wiesbaden: Franz Steiner, 1977.

Matheson, Lister M., ed. "John of Burgundy: Treatises on Plague." In *Sex, Aging, and Death in a Medieval Medical Compendium: Trinity College Cambridge MS R.14.52, Its Texts, Language, and Scribe*, edited by M. Teresa Tavormina, 569–602. Tempe, AZ: Arizona Center for Medieval and Renaissance Studies, 2006.

Nicholas of Lynn. *The Kalendarium of Nicholas of Lynn*, edited by Sigmud Eisner. Athens, GA: University of Georgia Press, 1980.

Oribasius. *Oeuvres d'Oribase*, edited by U.C. Bussemaker, Charles Daremberg, and Auguste Molinier, 6 vols. Paris, 1873–6.

Petrus Alfonsi. *The Disciplina Clericalis of Petrus Alfonsi*, edited by Eberhard Hermes. London: Routledge and Kegan Paul, 1977.

Petrus Hispanus. *Obras medicas de P. Hispano*, edited by M.H. da Rocha Pereira. Coimbra: Universidade, 1973.

Platearius. *Das Arzneidrogenbuch Circa instans in einer Fassung des XIII. Jahrhunderts aus der Universitätsbibliothek Erlangen*, ed. Hans Wölfel (Diss. Friedrich-Wilhelms-Universität, Berlin), 1939.

Somer, John. *The Kalendarium of John Somer*, edited by Linne R. Mooney. Athens, GA: University of Georgia Press, 1998.

Stoffregen, M., ed. "Eine frühmittelalterliche lateinische Übersetzung des byzantinischen Puls- und Urintraktats des Alexandros." PhD diss., Freie Universität Berlin, 1977.

Tavormina, M. Teresa, ed. *The Dome of Uryne: A Reading Edition of Nine Middle English Uroscopies*. EETS o.s. 354. Oxford: Oxford University Press, 2019.

– "The Twenty-Jordan Series: An Illustrated Middle English Uroscopy Text." *ANQ* 18, no. 3 (2005): 40–64.

Theophilus. *Liber urinarum a uoce Theophili. Edition einer Übersetzung des 12. Jahrhunderts mit ausführlichem Glossar*, edited by Sonya Dase. Marburg: Tectum Verlag, 1999.

– *Physici et medici Graeci minores* vol. 1, edited by Julius Ludwig Ideler. Berlin: Reimer; rpt. Amsterdam: Adolf M. Hakkert, 1963 and Angeletti, Cavarra and Gazzaniga, (1841) 1999.

Trevisa, John. *On the Properties of Things: John Trevisa's Translation of Bartholomaeus Anglicus De proprietatibus rerum: A Critical Text*. 3 vols., edited by M.C. Seymour (gen. ed.) et al. Oxford: Clarendon Press, 1975–1988.

– "Trevisa's Original Prefaces on Translation: a Critical Edition," edited by Ronald Waldron. In *Medieval English Studies Presented to George Kane*, edited by Edward Donald Kennedy, Ronald Waldron, and Joseph S. Wittig, 285–99. Suffolk: D.S. Brewer, 1988.

## Secondary Sources

Agrimi, Jole, and Chiara Crisciani. "Per una ricerca su 'Experimentum-experimenta': riflessione epistemological e tradizione medica (secoli XIII–XV)." In *Presenza del lessico greco e latino nelle lingue contemporanee: ciclo di lezioni tenute all'Universita do Macerate nell'a.a. 1987–88*, edited by Pietro Janni and Innocenzo Mazzini, 9–49. Macerata: Universita di Macerata, 1990.

– "The Science and Practice of Medicine in the Thirteenth Century According to Guglielmo da Saliceto, Italian Surgeon." In *Practical Medicine from Salerno to the Black Death*, edited by Luis Garcia-Ballester, Roger French, Jon Arrizabalaga, and Andrew Cunningham, 60–87. Cambridge: Cambridge University Press, 1994.

Akbari, Suzanne Conklin. *Seeing Through the Veil: Optical Theory and Medieval Allegory*. Toronto: University of Toronto Press, 2004.

Angeletti, Luciana Rita and Bernice Cavarra. "Critical and Historical Approach to Theophilus' *De urinis*. Urine as Blood's Percolation made by the Kidney and Uroscopy in the Middle Ages." *American Journal of Nephrology* 14 (1994): 282–9.

Angeletti, Luciana Rita, and Valentina Gazzaniga. "Theophilus' *Auctoritas*: The Role of *De urinis* in the Medical Curriculum of the 12th and 13th Centuries." *American Journal of Nephrology* 19 (1999): 165–71.

Ausécache, Mireille. "Gilles de Corbeil ou le médecin pédagogique au tournant des XIIe et XIIIe siècles," *Early Science and Medicine* 3 (1998): 187–215.

– "Introduction." In *Liber de uirtutibus et laudibus compositorum medicaminum*, edited by Mireille Ausécache. Florence: SISMEL/Edizioni del Galluzzo, 2017.

Beck, R. Theodore. *The Cutting Edge: Early History of the Surgeons of London.* London: Lund Humphries, 1974.

Black, Winston. "Henry of Huntingdon's Lapidary Rediscovered and his *Anglicanus Ortus* Reassembled." *Mediaeval Studies* 68 (2006): 43–87.

– "Review: Ulrike Jansen, '*Spuria Macri*': Ein Anhang zu '*Macer Floridus, De viribus herbarum.*' Einleitung, Übersetzung, Kommentar." *Speculum* 90, no. 1 (2015): 260–3.

– "Scenes from an Anglo-Norman Kitchen, Part 1: Mutton, Parsley, and Pagan Gods." *The Recipe Project* Oct. 13, 2016, https://recipes.hypotheses.org/8550.

– "Scenes from an Anglo-Norman Kitchen, Part 2: Vegetable Cures and a Drunken Cook." *The Recipe Project* 3 Nov. 2016, https://recipes.hypotheses.org/8588.

– "Teaching the Mnemonic Bishop in the Medieval Canon Law Classroom." In *Envisioning the Bishop: Images and the Episcopacy in the Middle Ages*, edited by Evan Gatti and Sigrid Danielson, 377–404. Turnhout: Brepols, 2014.

Bouras-Vallianatos, Petros. *Innovation in Byzantine Medicine: The Writings of John Zacharias Aktouarios (c. 1275–c. 1330).* Oxford: Oxford University Press, 2020. 69–103.

Brewer, Charlotte. *Editing Piers Plowman: The Evolution of the Text.* Cambridge: Cambridge University Press, 1996.

Brewer, D.S. "The Relationship of Chaucer to the English and European Traditions." In *Chaucer and Chaucerians: Critical Studies in Middle English Literature*, edited by D.S. Brewer, 1–38. London: Nelson, 1966.

Burnett, Charles. "The Legend of Constantine the African." In *The Medieval Legends of Philosophers and Scholars* = Micrologus 21, 277–94. Florence: SISMEL/Edizioni del Galluzzo, 2013.

Burnley, J.D. *A Guide to Chaucer's Language.* Norman: University of Oklahoma Press, 1983.

Burrow, John A. "The Third Eye of Prudence." In *Medieval Futures: Attitudes to the Future in the Middle Ages*, edited by J.A. Burrow and Ian P. Wei, 37–48. Woodbridge: Boydell Press, 2000.

Bynum, Caroline Walker. *Wonderful Blood: Theology and Practice in Late Medieval Northern Germany and Beyond.* Philadelphia: University of Pennsylvania Press, 2007.

Cannon, Christopher. *The Grounds of English Literature*. Oxford: Oxford University Press, 2004.

– *The Making of Chaucer's English: A Study of Words*. Cambridge: Cambridge University Press, 1998.

Carey, Hilary M. *Courting Disaster: Astrology at the English Court and University in the Later Middle Ages*. London: MacMillan, 1992.

Cavarra, Berenice. "Medicine and Uroscopy, from IVth Cent. BC to VII AD." In *Il De urinis di Teofilo Protospatario: centralità di un segno clinic*. Medicina nei secoli, n.s. suppl., edited by Luciana Rita Angeletti, Berenice Cabarro, and Valentina Gazzaniga, 191–216. Rome: Casa editrice Università La Sapienza, 2009.

– "The *De urinis* of Theophilus." In *Il De urinis di Teofilo Protospatario: centralità di un segno clinic*. Medicina nei secoli, n.s. suppl., edited by Luciana Rita Angeletti, Berenice Cabarro, and Valentina Gazzaniga, 217–23. Rome: Casa editrice Università La Sapienza, 2009.

Chandelier, Joël. *Avicenne et la médecine en Italie: le Canon dans les universités (1200–1350)*. Paris: Champion, 2017.

Clarke, C.A.M. "Overhearing Complaint and the Dialectic of Consolation in Chaucer's Verse." *Reading Medieval Studies* 29 (2003): 19–30.

Cooper, Lisa H. "'His guttys wer out shake': Illness and Indigence in Lydgate's *Letter to Gloucester* and *Fabula duorum mercatorum*" *Studies in the Age of Chaucer* 30 (2008): 303–34.

Cooper, Lisa H., and Andrea Denny-Brown. *Lydgate Matters: Poetry and Material Culture in the Fifteenth Century*. New York: Palgrave Macmillan, 2008.

Copeland, Rita. *Pedagogy, Intellectuals, and Dissent in the Later Middle Ages: Lollardy and Ideas of Learning*. Cambridge: Cambridge University Press, 2001.

Creutz, R. "Die Ehrenrettung Konstantins von Afrika." *Studien und Mitteilungen des Benediktiner Ordens* 49: 40–1; translated by Faith Wallis, (1931) 2010.

Crisciani, Chiara. "Histories, Stories, Exempla, and Anecdotes: Michele Savonarola from Latin to Vernacular." In *Historia: Empiricism and Erudition in Early Modern Europe*, edited by Gianna Pomata and Nancy G. Siraisi, 297–324. Cambridge, MA: MIT Press, 2005.

Crowcroft, Kathryn. "Reconsidering Sense: Towards a Theory of Medieval Preventative Medicine." *Postmedieval: A Journal of Medieval Cultural Studies* 8, no. 2 (2017): 162–9.

Daly, Walter J., and Robert D. Yee. "The Eye Book of Master Peter of Spain – A Glimpse of Diagnosis and Treatment of Eye Disease in the Middle Ages." *Documenta Ophthalmologica* 103 (2001): 119–53.

Demaitre, Luke. *Medieval Medicine: The Art of Healing, from Head to Toe*. Santa Barbara, CA: Praeger, 2013.

Denifle, H., and E. Chatelain. *Cartularium Universitatis Parisiensis*. Paris: Delalaine, 1889–97.

Dimitriadis, K. "Byzantinische Uroskopie." PhD diss., Bonn: Universität Bonn, 1971.

Ebin, Lois A. *Illuminator, Makar, Vates: Visions of Poetry in the Fifteenth Century*. Lincoln and London: University of Nebraska Press, 1988.

Emden, A.B. *A Biographical Register of the University of Oxford to A.D. 1500*. Oxford: Clarendon Press, 1957.

Espie, Jeff. "Literary Paternity and Narrative Revival: Chaucer's Souls from Spenser to Dryden." *Modern Philology* 114 (2016): 39–58.

– "(Un)couth: Chaucer, *The Shepheardes Calender*, and the Forms of Mediation." *Spenser Studies* 31 (2017): 243–71.

*eTK*. A digital resource based on Lynn Thorndike and Pearl Kibre, *A Catalogue of Incipits of Mediaeval Scientific Writings in Latin* (Cambridge, MA: Medieval Academy, 1963) and supplements, 2017. https://cctr1.umkc.edu/search.

– Expanded and revised version of Linda Ehrsam Voigts and Patricia Deery Kurtz, *Scientific and Medical Writings in Old and Middle English: An Electronic Reference*, 2014. https://cctr1.umkc.edu/search.

French, Roger. *Canonical Medicine: Gentile da Foligno and Scholasticism*. Leiden: Brill, 2001.

Gasper, Giles, and Faith Wallis. "Anselm and the *Articella*." *Traditio* 59 (2004): 129–74.

Gazzaniga, Valentina "Urology and Uroscopy from Hippocrates to Roman Medicine." In *Il De urinis di Teofilo Protospatario: centralità di un segno clinic*. Medicina nei secoli, n.s. suppl., edited by Luciana Rita Angeletti, Berenice Cabarro, and Valentina Gazzaniga, 175–89. Rome: Casa editrice Università La Sapienza, 2009.

Geaman, Kristen L. "Anne of Bohemia and Her Struggle to Conceive." *Social History of Medicine* 29, no. 2 (2016): 224–44.

Getz, Faye Marie. "Charity, Translation, and the Language of Medical Learning in Medieval England." *Bulletin of the History of Medicine* 64 (1990): 1–17.

– "The Faculty of Medicine before 1500." In *The History of the University of Oxford*, Vol.2, *Late Medieval Oxford*, edited by Jeremy Catto and Ralph Evans, 373–405. Oxford: Oxford University Press, 1992.

– "John Mirfield and the Breviarium Bartholomei: The Medical Writings of a Clerk at St Bartholomew's Hospital in the Later Fourteenth Century." *Society for the Social History of Medicine Bulletin* 37 (1985): 24–6.

– *Medicine in the English Middle Ages*. Princeton, NJ: Princeton University Press, 1998.

– "Medieval Practitioners in Medieval England." *Social History of Medicine* 3 (1990): 245–83.

Glick, Thomas F., Steven John Livesy, and Faith Wallis, eds. *Medieval Science, Technology, and Medicine: An Encyclopedia*. New York: Routledge, 2005.

Green, Monica H. *Making Women's Medicine Masculine: The Rise of Male Authority in Pre-Modern Gynaecology*. Oxford: Oxford University Press, 2008.

– "Medical Books." In *The European Book in the Twelfth Century*, edited by Erik Kwakkel and Rodney Thomson, 277–92. Cambridge: Cambridge University Press, 2018.

– "Medicine in France and England in the Long Twelfth Century: Inheritors and Creators of European Medicine." In *France et Angleterre: manuscrits médiévaux entre 700 et 1200*, edited by Francesco Siri and Charlotte Noel, 365–90. Turnhout: Brepols, 2020.

– "Rethinking the Manuscript Basis of Salvatore De Renzi's *Collectio Salernitana*: The Corpus of Medical Writings in the 'Long' Twelfth Century." In *La* Collectio Salernitana *di Salvatore De Renzi*, edited by Danielle Jacquart and Agostino Paravicini Bagliana, 15–60. Florence: SISMEL/Edizioni del Galluzzo, 2008.

Green, Richard Firth. "Friar William Appleton and the Date of Langland's B Text." *The Yearbook of Langland Studies* 11 (1997): 87–96.

Hanna, Ralph. *Pursuing History: Middle English Manuscripts and Their Texts*. Stanford: Stanford University Press, 1996.

Hanna, Ralph, ed. "Henry Daniel's *Liber Uricrisiarum*, Book I, Chapters 1–3." In *Popular and Practical Science of Medieval England*, edited Lister M. Matheson, 185–218. East Lansing, MI: Colleagues Press, 1994.

Hardingham, Glenn James. "The Regimen in Late Medieval England." PhD diss., University of Cambridge, 2005.

Hartley, Percival Horton-Smith, and Harold Richard Aldridge. *Johannes de Mirfeld of St Bartholomew's, Smithfield: His Life and Works*. Cambridge: Cambridge University Press, 1936.

Harvey, E. Ruth. "Medicine and Science in Chaucer's Day." In *The Oxford Handbook of Chaucer*, edited by Suzanne Conklin Akbari and James Simpson, 440–55. Oxford: Oxford University Press, 2020.

– Unpublished study. *The Faithful Messenger: Urine and Uroscopy in the Middle Ages*.

Hudson, Anne. "The Debate on Bible Translation, Oxford 1401," *English Historical Review* XC, CCCLIV (1975): 1–18.

– *The Premature Reformation: Wycliffite Texts and Lollard History*. Oxford: Clarendon Press, 1988.

Humphreys, Kenneth William. *The Friars' Libraries*. Corpus of British Medieval Library Catalogues 1. London: British Library in association with the British Academy, 1990.

Hunt, Tony. *Plant Names of Medieval England*. Cambridge: D.S. Brewer, 1989.

Iorio, Luigi, and Faustino Avagliano. "Observations on the *Liber medicine orinalibus* by Hermogenes." *American Journal of Nephrology* 19, no. 2 (1999): 185–8.

Jansen, Ulrike. *"Spuria Macri": Ein Anhang zu "Macer Floridus, De viribus herbarum." Einleitung, Übersetzung, Kommentar.* Berlin: De Gruyter, 2013.

Jacquart, Danielle. "La place d'Isaac Israeli dans la médicine médiévale," *Veslius* special number: 19–27, 1998.

– "La réception du Canon d'Avicenne: comparaison entre Montpellier et Paris au XIIIe et XIVe siècles." In *Histoire de l'École médicale de Montpellier. Actes du 110e Congrès national des Sociétés savantes (Montpellier 1985)*, 68–77. Paris: C.T.H.S. vol. 2, 1985.

– "Le regard d'un médecin sur son temps: Jacques Despars (1380?-1458)." *Bibliothèque de l'École des chartes* 138 (1980): 35–86.

– "Theory, Everyday Practice, and Three Fifteenth-Century Physicians." *Osiris* 6 (1990): 140–61.

Jacquart, Danielle, and Agostino Paravicini Bagliani, eds. *La* Collectio Salernitana *di Salvatore De Renzi: convegno internazionale, Università degli studi di Salerno.* Florence: SISMEL/Edizioni del Galluzzo, 2008.

Jacquart, Danielle, and Agostino Paravicini Bagliani, eds. *La Scuola Medica Salernitana. Gli autori e i testi.* Florence: SISMEL/Edizioni del Galluzzo, 2007.

Jacquart, Danielle, and Françoise Micheau. *La médecine arabe et l'occident médiéval.* Paris: Maisonneuve & Larose, 1990.

Jasin, Joanne. "The Transmission of Learned Medical Literature in the Middle English *Liber Uricrisiarum*." *Medical History* 37 (1993): 313–29.

Jones, Lori. "Bubo Men/*Pest-Aderlaßmann*? Repurposing Fifteenth- and Sixteenth-Century Therapeutic Anatomical Illustrations for the Plague." In *Death and Disease in the Medieval and Early Modern World: Perspectives from Across the Mediterranean and Beyond*, edited by Lori Jones and Nükhet Varlik. Woodbridge, Suffolk: York Medieval Press. Forthcoming.

Jones, Peter Murray. "Alchemical Remedies in Late Medieval England." In *Alchemy and Medicine from Antiquity to the Enlightenment*, edited by Jennifer Rampling and Peter Murray Jones. Abingdon-on-Thames: Routledge, 2017.

– "Complexio and Experimentum: Tensions in Late Medieval Medical Practice." In *The Body in Balance: Humoral Medicines in Practice*, edited by Peregrine Horden and Elisabeth Hus, 107–28. New York: Berghahn Books, 2013.

– "Harley MS 2558: a Fifteenth-Century Medical Commonplace Book." In *Manuscript Sources of Medieval Medicine: A Book of Essays*, edited by Margaret R. Schleissner, 35–54. New York, London: Garland, 1995.

– "John Arderne and the Mediterranean Tradition of Scholastic Surgery." In *Practical Medicine from Salerno to the Black Death*, edited by Luis Garcia-Ballester, Roger French, Jon Arrizabalaga and Andrew Cunningham, 289–321. Cambridge: Cambridge University Press, 1994.

- "Language and Register in English Medieval Surgery." In *Language in Medieval Britain: Networks and Exchanges: Proceedings of the 2013 Harlaxton Symposium*, edited by Mary Carruthers, 74–89. Donington: Shaun Tyas, 2015.
- "Mediating Collective Experience: The *Tabula Medicine* (1416–1425) as a Handbook for Medical Practice." In *Between Text and Patient: The Medical Enterprise in Medieval and Early Modern Europe*, Micrologus' Library 39, edited by Florence Eliza Glaze and Brian K. Nance, 279–307. Florence: SISMEL/Edizioni del Galluzzo, 2011.
- "The Surgeon as Story-Teller." *Poetica (An International Journal of Linguistic-Literary Studies)* 72 (2009): 77–91.
- "The Survival of the Frater Medicus? English Friars and Alchemy, 1370–1425." *Ambix* 65, no. 3 (2018): 232–49.
- "The '*Tabula medicine*': An Evolving Encyclopedia." In *English Manuscript Studies, 1100–1700*, volume 14, *Regional Manuscripts, 1200–1700*, edited by A.S.G. Edwards, 60–85. London: British Library, 2008.
- "Thomas Fayreford: An English Fifteenth-Century Medical Practitioner." In *Medicine from the Black Death to the French Disease*, edited by Roger French, Jon Arrizabalaga, Andrew Cunningham and Luis Garcia-Ballester, 156–83. Aldershot: Ashgate, 1998.
Kean, P.M. *Chaucer and the Making of English Poetry: The Art of Narrative.* London and Boston: Routledge and Kegan Paul, 1972.
Keil, Gundolf. *Die urognostische Praxis in Vor- und Frühsalernitanischer Zeit.* Habilitationsschrift, Albert-Ludwigs-Universität, Freiburg im Breisgau, 1970.
Keiser, George R. *A Manual of the Writings in Middle English 1050–1500*, Vol. 10 *Works of Science and Information.* New Haven: Connecticut Academy of Arts and Sciences, 1998.
- "Rosemary: Not Just for Remembrance." In *Health and Healing from the Medieval Garden*, edited by Peter Dendle and Alain Touwaide, 180–204. Woodbridge: Boydell, 2008.
- "Vernacular Herbals: A Growth Industry in Late Medieval England." In *Design and Distribution of Late Medieval Manuscripts in England*, edited by Margaret Connolly and Linne R. Mooney, 292–308. Woodbridge: York Medieval Press, 2008.
Ker, Neil Ripley, ed. *Medieval Libraries of Great Britain: A List of Surviving Books.* Second Edition. London: Royal Historical Society, 1964.
Kristeller, Paul Oskar. "Bartholomaeus, Musandinus and Maurus of Salerno and other Early Commentators of the Articella, with a Tentative List of Texts and Manuscripts." *Italia medioevale e umanistica* 29: 57–87; translated 1986: "Bartolomeo, Musandino, Mauro di Salerno e altri antichi commentatori dell'*Articella*, con un elenco di testi e di manoscritti." In *Studi sulla scuola*

*medica salernitana*, 97–151. Naples: Istituto italiano per gli studi filosofici, 1976.

*LALME*. See McIntosh et al.

Lang, Sheila J. "John Bradmore and his book *Philomena.*" *Social History of Medicine* 5 (1992): 121–30.

– "John Bradmore and the Case of the Bitten Man: A Tantalising Link Between Three Medieval Surgical Manuscripts." *Social History of Medicine*, hkaa014, 2020. https://doi.org/10.1093/shm/hkaa014.

Law, Vivien. "Why Write a Verse Grammar?" *Journal of Medieval Latin* 9 (1999): 46–76.

Lerer, Seth. *Chaucer and His Readers: Imagining the Author in Late Medieval England.* Princeton, NJ: Princeton University Press, 1993.

Lloyd, G.E.R. "Galen's Un-Hippocratic Case-Histories." In *Galen and the World of Knowledge*, edited by Christopher Gill, Tim Whitmarsh, and John Wilkins, 115–31. Cambridge: Cambridge University Press, 2009.

Mäkinen, Martti. "Henry Daniel's Rosemary in MS X.90 of the Royal Library, Stockholm." *Neuphilologische Mitteilungen* 103, no. 3 (2002): 305–27.

– "Herbal recipes and recipes in herbals – intertextuality in early English medical writing." In *Medical and Scientific Writing in Late Medieval English*, edited by Irma Taavitsainen and Päivi Pahta, 144–73. Cambridge: Cambridge University Press, 2004.

Mann, Jill. *Chaucer and Medieval Estates Satire: The Literature of Social Classes and the General Prologue to The Canterbury Tales.* Cambridge: Cambridge University Press, 1973.

Matheson, Lister M., ed. *Popular and Practical Science of Medieval England.* East Lansing, MI: Colleagues Press, 1994.

Maxwell-Stuart, P.G. *Studies in Greek Colour Terminology.* Leiden: Brill, 1981.

McFarlane, K.B. "William Worcester: A Preliminary Survey." In *Studies Presented to Sir Hilary Jenkinson*, edited by J. Conway Davies, 196–221. London: Oxford University Press, 1957.

McIntosh, Angus, Michael L. Samuels, and Michael Benskin. *A Linguistic Atlas of Late Mediaeval English.* 4 vols. Aberdeen: Aberdeen University Press [*LALME*]. Rev. and supp. by Michael Benskin, Margaret Laing, Vasilis Karaiskos, and Keith Williamson. 2013. *An Electronic Version of A Linguistic Atlas of Late Mediaeval English.* Edinburgh: University of Edinburgh, 1986. http://www.lel.ed.ac.uk/ihd/elalme/elalme.html [*eLALME*].

McKitterick, Rosamond, and Richard Beadle. *Catalogue of the Pepys Library at Magdalene College, Cambridge.* Vol. v, part 1: Manuscripts, Medieval. Cambridge: Brewer, 1992.

McVaugh, Michael R. "Bedside Manners in the Middle Ages." *Bulletin of the History of Medicine* 71 (1997): 201–23.

– "The Experimenta of Arnald of Villanova." *Journal of Medieval and Renaissance Studies* 1 (1971): 107–18.
– *The Rational Surgery of the Middle Ages*. Florence: SISMEL/Edizioni del Galluzzo, 2006.
– "Who was Gilbert the Englishman?" In *The Study of Medieval Manuscripts in England: Festschrift in Honor of Richard W. Pfaff*, edited by George Hardin Brown and Linda Ehrsam Voigts, 302–4. Tempe: Arizona Center for Medieval and Renaissance Studies in collaboration with Brepols, 2010.
Meyer, Heinz. *Die Enzyklopädie des Bartholomäus Anglicus. Untersuchungen zur Überlieferungs- und Rezeptionsgeschichte von "De proprietatibus rerum."* Munich: Wilhelm Fink, 2000.
Michael, Matthew. "Secret Talk and Eavesdropping Scenes: Its Literary Effects and Significance in Biblical Narrative." *Vetus Testamentum* 65, no. 1 (2015): 91–113.
*MLGB3* [Medieval Libraries of Great Britain]. 2015. http://mlgb3.bodleian.ox.ac.uk/.
Montford, Angela. *Health, Sickness, and the Friars in the Thirteenth and Fourteenth Centuries*. Aldershot: Ashgate, 2004.
Moulinier-Brogi, Laurence. *Guillaume l'Anglais, le frondeur de l'uroscopie médiévale (XIIIe siècle)*. Geneva: Droz, 2011.
– "La science des urines de Maurus de Salerne et les *Sinthomata Magistri Mauri* inédits." In *La Scuola medica Salernitana. Gli autori et I testi*, edited by Danielle Jacquart and Agostino Paravicini Bagliani, 261–81. Florence: SISMEL/Edizioni del Galluzzo, 2007.
– *L'Uroscopie au Moyen Âge. "Lire dans un verre la nature de l'homme."* Paris: Honoré Champion, 2012.
Newton, Francis, trans. "Die Ehrenrettung Konstantins von Afrika." In *Mediterranean Passages: Readings from Dido to Derrida*, edited by Miriam Cooke, Erdağ Göknar, and Grant Parker, 116–17. Chapel Hill: University of North Carolina Press, 2008.
North, John David. *Chaucer's Universe*. Oxford: Clarendon, 1988.
Norton-Smith, John. *John Lydgate: Poems*. Oxford: Clarendon Press, 1966.
O'Boyle, Cornelius. *Medieval Prognosis and Astrology. A Working Edition of the Aggregationes de crisi et creticis diebus: with Introduction and English Summary*. Cambridge: Wellcome Unit for the History of Medicine, 1991.
Olalla, David Moreno. *"The fautys to amende*: On the Interpretation of the *Explicit* of Sloane 5, ff. 13–57, and Related Matters." *English Studies* 88:2 (2007): 119–42.
Oldoni, Massimo. "Uroscopy in the Salerno School of Medicine." *American Journal of Nephrology* 14 (1994): 483–7.
Olsan, Lea T. "Charms and Prayers in Medieval Medical Theory and Practice." *Social History of Medicine* 16 (2003): 343–66.

O'Neill, Ynez Viole. "William of Conches' Descriptions of the Brain." *Clio Medica* 3 (1968): 203–23.

Orlemanski, Julie. *Symptomatic Subjects: Bodies, Medicine, and Causation in the Literature of Late Medieval England*. Pennsylvania: University of Pennsylvania Press, 2019.

*Oxford Dictionary of National Biography* [*ODNB*]. http://www.oxforddnb.com.

Pahta, Päivi, and Irma Taavitsainen. "Vernacularisation of scientific and medical writing in its sociohistorical context." In *Medical and Scientific Writing in Late Medieval English*, edited by Irma Taavitsainen and Päivi Pahta, 1–18, at 14. Cambridge University Press, 2004.

Pearsall, Derek. *John Lydgate*. London: Routledge and Kegan Paul, 1970.

Peine, Johannes. "Die Harnschrift des Isaac Judaeus." PhD diss., Leipzig MD, 1919.

Peterson, D.W. 1974. "Galen's 'Therapeutics to Glaucon' and its Early Commentaries." PhD diss., Johns Hopkins University, 1974.

Rand Schmidt, Kari Anne. *Manuscripts in the Library of Gonville and Caius College, Cambridge*. Index of Middle English Prose, Handlist 17. Cambridge: Brewer, 2001.

Rider, Catherine. *Magic and Impotence in the Middle Ages*. Oxford: Oxford University Press, 2006.

Ronca, Italo. *Guillelmi de Conchis Dragmaticon philosophiae*. Turnhout: Brepols, 1997.

Rouse, Mary A., and Richard H. Rouse. *Authentic Witnesses: Approaches to Medieval Texts and Manuscripts*. Notre Dame, IN: University of Notre Dame Press, 1991.

Scanlon, Larry. *Narrative Authority and Power: The Medieval Exemplum and the Chaucerian Tradition*. Cambridge: Cambridge University Press, 1994.

Seaton, Ethel. *Sir Richard Roos, c. 1410–1482: Lancastrian Poet*. London: R. Hart-Davis, 1961.

Sharpe, Richard. *A Handlist of the Latin Writers of Great Britain and Ireland before 1540*. Turnhout: Brepols, 1997.

Sigerist, Henry E. "Bedside Manners in the Middle Ages: The Treatise *De cautelis medicorum* Attributed to Arnald of Villanova." *Quarterly Bulletin of the Northwest University Medical School* 20 (1946): 136–43.

Siraisi, Nancy. *Avicenna in Renaissance Italy: The Canon and Medical Teaching in Italian Universities after 1500*. Princeton: Princeton University Press, 1987.

– "Girolamo Cardano and the Art of Medical Narrative," *Journal of the History of Ideas* 52 (1991): 581–602.

– *Medicine and the Italian Universities, 1250–1600*. Leiden: Brill, 2001.

– *Taddeo Alderotti and his Pupils: Two Generations of Italian Medical Learning*. Princeton: Princeton University Press, 1981.

Somerset, Fiona. *Clerical Discourse and Lay Audience in Late Medieval England*. Cambridge: Cambridge University Press, 1998.

Star, Sarah. *"Anima Carnis in Sanguine Est*: Blood, Life, and *The King of Tars."* *JEGP* 115, no. 4 (2016): 442–62.

– "Henry Daniel, Medieval English Medicine, and Linguistic Innovation: A Lexicographic Study of Huntington MS HM 505," *Huntington Library Quarterly* 81, no. 1 (2018): 63–106.

– "The Textual Worlds of Henry Daniel." *Studies in the Age of Chaucer* 40 (2018): 191–216.

Sudhoff, Karl. "Commentatoren der Harnverse des Gilles de Corbeil." *Archeion* 11 (1929): 128–35.

Taavitsainen, Irma. "Transferring Classical Discourse Conventions into the Vernacular." In *Medical and Scientific Writing in Late Medieval English,* edited by Irma Taavitsainen and Päivi Pahta, 37–72. Cambridge: Cambridge University Press, 2004.

Talbot, Charles H. "Simon Bredon (c.1300–1372), Physician, Mathematician, and Astronomer." *British Journal for the History of Science* 1 (1962–3): 19–30.

Talbot, Charles H., and E.A. Hammond. *The Medical Practitioners in Medieval England: A Biographical Register.* London: Wellcome Historical Medical Library, 1965.

Tavormina, M. Teresa. "Uroscopy in Middle English: A Guide to the Texts and Manuscripts." *Studies in Medieval & Renaissance History.* 3rd series. 11 (2014): 1–154.

Tavormina, M. Teresa, ed. *Sex, Aging, and Death in a Medieval Medical Compendium: Trinity College Cambridge MS R.14.52, Its Texts, Language, and Scribe,* 2 vols. Tempe, AZ: Arizona Center for Medieval and Renaissance Studies, 2006.

Thomson, Rodney M. *A Descriptive Catalogue of the Medieval Manuscripts in the Library of Peterhouse, Cambridge.* Cambridge: D.S. Brewer, 2016.

Thorndike, Lynn. *The Sphere of Sacrobosco and its Commentators.* Corpus of mediaeval scientific texts, Mediaeval Academy of America and the University of Chicago, v. 2, 1949.

– "Unde Versus." *Traditio* 11 (1955): 163–93.

Thorndike, Lynn, and Pearl Kibre. *Incipits of Medieval Scientific Works in Latin.* Cambridge MA: Mediaeval Academy of America, 1963.

Turner, Marion. "Illness Narratives in the Later Middle Ages: Arderne, Chaucer and Hoccleve." *Journal of Medieval and Early Modern Studies* 46, no 1 (2016): 64–5.

Van der Lugt, Maaike. "'Abominable ixtures': The 'Liber vaccae' in the Medieval West, or the Dangers and Attractions of Natural Magic." *Traditio,* 64 (2009): 229–77.

Veit, Raphaela. *Das Buch der Fieber des Isaac Israeli und seine Bedeutung im lateinischen Westen: ein Beitrag zur Rezeption arabischer Wissenschaft im Abendland,* Sudhoffs Archiv Beiheft 51. Stuttgart: Franz Steiner, 2003.

– "Quellenkundliches zu Leben und Werk von Constantinus Africanus." *Deutsches Archiv für Erforschung des Mittelalters* 59 (2003): 121–52.

Vieillard, Camille. *Essai sur la société médicale et religieuse au XIIe siècle: Gilles de Corbeil* .... Paris: Honoré Champion, 1909.

– *L'Urologie et les médecins urologues dans la médecine ancienne: Gilles de Corbeil, sa vie, ses oeuvres, son poème des urines.* Paris: Rudeval, 1903.

Voigts, Linda Ehrson. "The Medical Astrology of Ralph Hoby, Fifteenth Century Franciscan." In *The Friars in Medieval Britain: Proceedings of the 2007 Harlaxton Symposium,* edited by Nicholas Rogers, 152–68. Donington: Shaun Tyas, 2010.

– "Multitudes of Middle English Manuscripts, or the Englishing of Science and Medicine." In *Manuscript Sources of Medieval England: A Book of Essays,* edited by Margaret R. Schleissner, 183–96. New York and London: Garland Publishing, 1995.

– "Plants and Planets: Linking the Vegetable with the Celestial in Late Medieval Texts." In *Health and Healing from the Medieval Garden,* edited by Peter Dendle and Alain Touwaide, 29–46. Woodbridge: Boydell, 2008.

– "Scientific and Medical Books." In *Book Production and Publishing in Britain, 1375–1475,* edited by Jeremy Griffiths and Derek Pearsall, 345–402. Cambridge: Cambridge University Press, 1989.

– "Wolfenbüttel HAB Cod. Guelf. 51. 9. Aug. 4° and BL, Harley MS. 3542: Complementary Witnesses to Ralph Hoby's 1437 Treatise on Astronomical Medicine." *Electronic British Library Journal.* Article 10.

Voigts, Linda E., and Michael R. McVaugh. *A Latin Technical Phlebotomy and Its Middle English Translation.* Transactions of the American Philosophical Society 74, no. 2 (1984). Philadelphia: American Philosophical Society.

Voigts, Linda Ehrsam, and Patricia Deery Kurtz. *Scientific and Medical Writings in Old and Middle English: An Electronic Reference,* rev. ed., 2014. http://www.medievalacademy.org/?page=DigitalTools [eVK2].

Walling, Amanda. "Feminizing Aureation in Lydgate's *Life of Our Lady* and *Life of Saint Margaret.*" *Neophilologus* 101, no. 2 (2017): 321–36.

Wallis, Faith. "The *Articella* Commentaries of Magister Bartholomaeus." In *La Scuola Medica Salernitana: gli autori e i testi,* edited by Danielle Jacquart and Agostino Paravicini Bagliani, 125–64. Florence: SISMEL/Edizioni del Galluzzo, 2007.

– "The Experience of the Book: Manuscripts, Texts, and the Role of Epistemology in Early Medieval Medicine." In *Knowledge and the Scholarly Medical Traditions,* edited by Don G. Bates, 101–26. Cambridge: Cambridge University Press, 1995.

– "Inventing Diagnosis: Theophilus' *De urinis* in the Classroom." *Dynamis* 20 (2000): 31–73.

– "Signs and Senses: Diagnosis and Prognosis in Early Medieval Pulse and Urine Texts." *Social History of Medicine* 13, no. 2 (2000): 265–78.

- "Why was the Aphorisms of Hippocrates Re-Translated in the Eleventh Century?" In *Vehicles of Transmission, Translation and Transformation*, edited by Carlos Fraenkel, Jamie Fumo, Faith Wallis, and Robert Wisnovsky, 179–99. Turnhout: Brepols, 2011.
- ed. *Medieval Medicine: A Reader*, 138–9. Toronto: University of Toronto Press, 1931.
Walsh Morrissey, Jake. "Anxious Love and Disordered Urine: The Englishing of *Amor Hereos* in Henry Daniel's *Liber uricrisiarum*." *Chaucer Review* 49, no. 2 (2014): 161–83.
Walter, Katie L. "The Form of the Formless: Medieval Taxonomies of Skin, Flesh, and the Human." In *Reading Skin in Medieval Literature and Culture*, edited by Katie L. Walter, 119–39. New York: Palgrave Macmillan, 2013.
White, Hayden. "The Value of Narrativity in the Representation of Reality." *Critical Inquiry* 7, no. 1 (1980): 5–27.
Whiting, Bartlett Jere. *Proverbs, Sentences, and Proverbial Phrases from English Writings mainly before 1500*. Cambridge, MA: Harvard University Press, 1968.
Ziolkowski, Jan. "From Didactic Poetry to Bestselling Textbooks in the Long Twelfth Century." In *Calliope's Classroom: Studies in Didactic Poetry from Antiquity to the Renaissance*, edited by Annette Harder, Alasdair A. MacDonald, and Gerrit J. Reinink, 221–44. Leuven: Peeters, 2007.

# Contributors

**Winston Black** is the Gatto Chair of Christian Studies at St. Francis Xavier University in Antigonish, Nova Scotia. He is a historian of medicine, science, and theology in the High Middle Ages, with a focus on England and France. He published an edition, translation, and study of Henry of Huntingdon's *Anglicanus Ortus: A Verse Herbal of the Twelfth Century* (2012), which Henry Daniel used as a key source in his own herbal. He is the author of *Medicine and Healing in the Premodern West* (2019), *The Middle Ages: Facts and Fictions* (2019), and *Medieval Herbalism and Pharmacy: A Case Study* (forthcoming). He is also a coauthor, with John M. Riddle, of *A History of the Middle Ages, 300–1500, Second Edition* (2016).

**Hannah Bower** is a Junior Research Fellow at Churchill College, Cambridge. Her research focuses on the boundaries, overlaps, and exchanges between literary writing and other, apparently practical or scientific genres. Her doctoral work on the linguistic and imaginative connections between medieval medical recipes and more canonical literary texts was funded by the Wellcome Trust. She also completed a six-month Wellcome secondment fellowship at the London Science Museum which explored the editorial history and reader reception of eighteenth-century medical pamphlets. Her current research continues this interdisciplinary approach by investigating the representation of human-engineered spectacles in all kinds of medieval writing and by exploring the role of *impossibilia* in creative, scientific, philosophical, and practical thought.

**E. Ruth Harvey** is a Professor Emerita at the Centre for Medieval Studies, University of Toronto. She is the author of *The Inward Wits: Psychological Theory in the Middle Ages and the Renaissance* (1975), and the editor of *The Court of Sapience* (1984) and of *Liber Uricrisiarum: A Reading Edition* (2020). Her research interests include medieval and early Renaissance learning, literature, and the history of medicine. She has written articles and book chapters on topics ranging from scientific and medical writing in the age of Chaucer and animal symbolism in literature to the history and practice of uroscopy, and has unearthed the complex manuscript and textual traditions of Henry Daniel's two major encyclopaedic works and their intellectual roots.

**Peter Murray Jones** is Fellow Librarian at King's College, Cambridge, UK, and an Affiliate of the Department of History and Philosophy of Science, University of Cambridge. He is currently writing a book on friars and medicine in England, 1224 to 1538. This will investigate the role of friars as medical practitioners as well as their contributions as authors and compilers of medical texts. His published work on medical history has centred on the relationship of knowledge to practice in late medieval and early modern England. This includes studies on the fourteenth-century English surgeon John Arderne, and on fifteenth-century medical practitioners who wrote about their own case-histories, like Thomas Fayreford and John Argentine. Language in medical and surgical writings is another focus of interest. He is a Principal Investigator on the Generation to Reproduction project in HPS, Cambridge. A biography of John Arderne is under contract.

**Sarah Star** is a Visiting Assistant Professor in the Department of English at Kenyon College. With E. Ruth Harvey and M. Teresa Tavormina, she is an editor of *Liber Uricrisiarum: A Reading Edition* (2020). Her work on topics such as Henry Daniel, vernacular medicine, medieval physiology, and literary representations of embodied identity has appeared in *Studies in the Age of Chaucer*, *The Journal of Medieval Religious Cultures*, and *JEGP*, among other venues. She is currently completing her first monograph, which focuses on the intersections of medieval medicine and literature, the symbolic valences of blood, and the significance of embodied religious identities.

**M. Teresa Tavormina** is a Professor Emerita in the Department of English, Michigan State University. Her publications and editorial work include *Kindly Similitude: Marriage and Family in Piers Plowman* (1995); *The Yearbook of Langland Studies*; *Medieval England: An Encyclopedia* (1998); *The Endless Knot: Studies in Old and Middle English Literature in Honor of Marie Borroff* (1995); *Sex, Aging, and Death in a Medieval Medical Compendium: Trinity College Cambridge MS R.14.52, Its Texts, Language,* *and Scribe* (2006); "Uroscopy in Middle English: A Guide to the Texts and Manuscripts" (*Studies in Medieval & Renaissance History*, ser. 3, vol. 11; 2014); *The Dome of Uryne: A Reading Edition of Nine Middle English Uroscopies* (Early English Text Society o.s. 354, 2020); *Liber Uricrisiarum: A Reading Edition* (2020); and shorter editions and articles on Chaucer, Langland, Middle English medical texts, science fiction, literature and medicine, and other topics.

**Faith Wallis** is a Professor jointly appointed in the Department of History and Classical Studies and the Department of Social Studies of Medicine at McGill University. Her research focuses on the transmission of medical and scientific knowledge in the Middle Ages. Her anthology of translated sources, *Medieval Medicine: A Reader*, was published in 2010. She has published editions and studies of Bede and Isidore of Seville, and articles and book chapters on medieval surgery, the translation and transmission of medical knowledge, herbals, and other medical topics. She is presently editing the writings of Bartholomeus "of Salerno," a key figure in the emergence of academic medicine in the twelfth century, and the full five-book version of *On the natures of things* (*De naturis rerum*) by the English scholar Alexander Neckam (d. 1217).

# Manuscript Index

# Index